Get Started

Pilates

Get Started

Pilates

LONDON, NEW YORK, MUNICH, MELBOURNE, DELHI

Project Editor Becky Shackleton
Project Art Editor Gemma Fletcher
Senior Editor Alastair Laing
Managing Editor Penny Warren
Managing Art Editor Alison Donovan
Senior Jacket Creative Nicola Powling
Jacket Design Assistant Rosie Levine
Pre-production Producer Sarah Isle
Producer Jen Lockwood
Art Directors Peter Luff, Jane Bull
Publisher Mary Ling

DK Inc
Editor Nichole Altorfer
Senior Editor Shannon Beatty

DK India
Editors Vibha Malhotra, Arani Sinha
Art Editors Ranjita Bhattacharji, Devan Das
DTP Manager Sunil Sharma
DTP Designers Sourabh Challariya, Arjinder Singh

Tall Tree Ltd
Editor Emma Marriott
Designer Ben Ruocco

Written by Anya Hayes

First American Edition, 2013

Published in the United States by DK Publishing,
375 Hudson Street, New York, New York 10014

10 9 8 7 6 5 4 3 2 1
001—187846—Jan/2013

Published in Great Britain by Dorling Kindersley Limited.

A catalog record for this book is available from the
Library of Congress.

ISBN 978-1-4654-0199-1

DK books are available at special discounts when purchased in
bulk for sales promotions, premiums, fund-raising, or educational
use. For details, contact: DK Publishing Special Markets, 375
Hudson Street, New York, New York 10014 or
SpecialSales@dk.com.

Printed and bound by Leo Paper Products Ltd, China

Discover more at
www.dk.com

Contents

Build Your Course 6 • Principles of Pilates 8 • Benefits of Pilates 12 • Essential Equipment 24
The Science of... Anatomy 18 • Alignment 20 • Breathing 22

Start Simple

Build On It

Take It Further

PUBLISHER'S NOTE
Neither the publisher nor the author is engaged in rendering professional advice or services to the individual reader. The ideas, procedures, and suggestions contained in this book are not intended as a substitute for consulting with your physician. All matters regarding your health require medical supervision. Neither the author nor the publisher shall be liable or responsible for any loss or damage allegedly arising from any information or suggestion in this book.

Build Your Course

This book is divided into three sections: Start Simple, Build On It, and Take It Further. As you progress through the book the positions gradually become more challenging and you will increase your physical ability, while also learning how to plan and assess your sessions.

Getting Started

In order to get the most from Pilates it is important to understand the ideas that underpin it. The introduction to this book guides you through the key principles of Pilates, from centring to breathing, and explains its benefits, which range from flexibility and alignment to toning and shaping. As well as delving a little deeper into the science of posture and breathing, it will show you the equipment you'll need.

1 In every section, illustrated step-by-step text guides you carefully through the exercises. The text explains in detail exactly how you need to position yourself.

Careful! To guide you and give further useful advice, key information about each step is flagged up, helping you to avoid common mistakes.

Pinpoints the exact places your body should be working

Highlights body parts to be aware of

Take care and Make it easier

It can be easy to think that you are performing an exercise correctly when in fact you're not. Some movements could strain your body if done incorrectly, so it's crucial not to make mistakes. The useful "Take care" boxes will teach you how to check and correct your posture, so you don't make common mistakes. Some boxes have illustrations so that you can clearly see how a movement should not be performed. If you are struggling with a difficult exercise, "Make it easier" boxes advise you how to modify the move so it's less of a strain.

Possible errors are flagged up

Planning and Assessing

It's important to plan your sessions so that you can set yourself goals and keep track of how hard you're working. It is also crucial to take a step back now and again to assess your progress and check that you aren't making any mistakes. At the beginning and end of each section are pages that will help you to create plans to reach specific goals, such as improving your centring or alignment, and pages that will help you to assess your progress (see the two examples below). They also answer common questions that you might have and offer helpful advice and guidance so you can achieve your goals.

Week 1: Focus on Alignment

Baseline: take photos of yourself standing – front, side, and back – and draw plumb lines on the images, as on pp.20–21.

- **Day 1:** 15-minute sequence, check scoop
- **Day 2:** 15-minute sequence, check lengthening
- **Day 3:** 15-minute sequence, check precision
- **Day 4:** 15-minute sequence, check stability
- **Day 5:** 15-minute sequence, check C-curve.

Goal: take new photos after six weeks to see how much closer you are to the ideal alignment.

Goal: Centring
Centring (see p.40)

Work on flowing movement from a strong core, keeping the spine still

Goal: Strength
Wall: Chair (see p.45), Hundred Preparation (see pp.54–55), Roll Up (see pp.58–59)

Work on staying stable through each exercise, flowing each one to the next without a break

---

Sequences

Once you've mastered the positions, the next step is to put them together and practise them as a sequence. At the end of each section is a selection of timed sequences for you to follow: choose from 15 , 30, and 45 minutes. The sequences give the names of the movements and their page references, so that you can flick back to check that you are doing them correctly.

1 **Pilates Stance** p.35

2 **Wall: Roll Down** pp.42–43

3 **Wall: Stand** p.44

The 6 Principles of Pilates

Joe Pilates based his body conditioning system on six principles. If you keep them in mind every time you work out, they will become second nature over time and your practice will be infinitely more effective. As Pilates said, these principles combine "to give you suppleness, natural grace, and skill."

1. Control

This is the most important principle from which all other Pilates principles stem. Joe Pilates's original name for his exercise system was Contrology. According to his philosophy, a few movements performed correctly—with complete muscular and mental control and purposeful, precise movement—were more effective than many repetitions performed sloppily. This applies to ALL movement, be it slow, swift, or dynamic. Control enables you to become more aware of where your body is in space and to work targeted muscles effectively.

Key points

- **Consider the execution** of every part of the movement. Control everything: alignment, breathing, pace, coordination.

- **Be certain about the exercise.** Memorize the breath pattern and movement so you can begin to control the entire exercise effectively. There should be no uncertainty in your movement.

- **Control the movement**: beginning, middle, and end. Always move with fluidity, strength, and precision. Never simply slump onto the mat at the end of a repetition.

How Joe developed Pilates: Joseph Pilates studied anatomy and trained as a body builder, gymnast, and boxer. He developed his exercise regime after the First World War in New York, where it was quickly taken up by ballet dancers as well as the city's elite. "Pilates Elders," who had trained directly with him, spread his work throughout the world. Some taught "classical" Pilates, exactly as he had taught them. Others developed the exercises in their own ways. Pilates continues to evolve today.

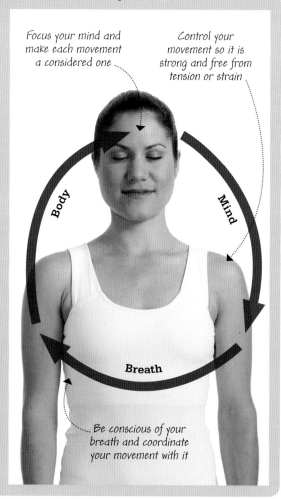

Focus your mind and make each movement a considered one

Control your movement so it is strong and free from tension or strain

Body

Mind

Breath

Be conscious of your breath and coordinate your movement with it

2. Concentration

Pilates requires deep focus on your body—as Joe Pilates said, "complete coordination of body, mind, and spirit." Your success in Pilates will hinge on your ability to concentrate on the precise detail of every movement, and so develop body awareness and control.

Be strict with yourself: Never let your mind wander or run on autopilot and perform mindless repetitions while you're working out. Always concentrate on the task at hand and your exercise will be much more effective and you will see results faster. This mental connection with your body allows you to release tension and encourages a deep sense of relaxation by emptying your mind of all other thoughts or worries.

Key points

- **Don't try to focus on the whole body** at once. Think about which muscles you're working, and focus on one part of your body or on your breathing. With practice, you'll be able to concentrate effectively on your whole body with ease.

- **Run through a checklist in your mind** as you work out. Think about lengthening parts of your body, how you breathe, and if you're engaging your powerhouse. Being your own teacher reaps great rewards.

- **Concentrate and correct yourself** as you move. Focus on perfecting the movement: notice if your alignment is off, if you have lost abdominal engagement, or if your neck is tense.

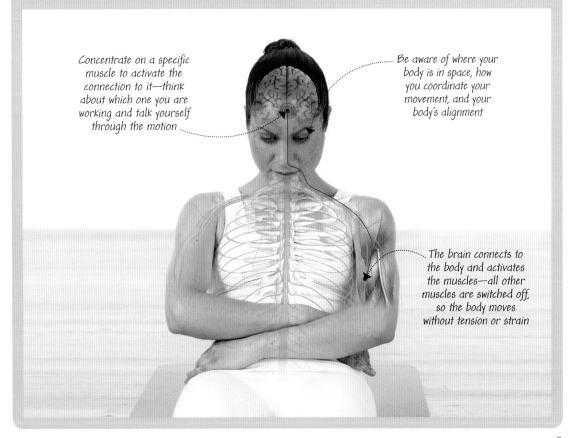

Concentrate on a specific muscle to activate the connection to it—think about which one you are working and talk yourself through the motion

Be aware of where your body is in space, how you coordinate your movement, and your body's alignment

The brain connects to the body and activates the muscles—all other muscles are switched off, so the body moves without tension or strain

3. Centering

Pilates taught that energy in movement "flows from a strong center." He noticed that drawing in the belly "navel to spine" tightened the muscles like a corset around his waist, supporting his spine and making it strong. He called this the "powerhouse" or "girdle of strength." Physically, the "center" is comprised of your core muscles: the pelvic floor and deep, lower abdominals. The powerhouse—including upper abdominals, buttocks, and inner-thigh muscles—provides strength for your movement. Centering also involves a mindful connection to your body as you move. Be aware of your center to begin and end each movement, so you never lose the connection.

A strong center means no needless tension elsewhere in the body

Engaging the center carries the leg's weight without compressing the lower back

The spine is stable and supported

Key points

- **Lift up your pelvic floor** and draw in the belly to tighten the powerhouse and create strength. Think "pull in and up."

- **Always pause briefly at the end** of a move to ensure your concentration and center connection are still strong.

- **Think of your center as a dimmer switch**: it is always on, but at different brightnesses. Turn it to full engagement for very hard work, or to low engagement for basic exercises.

4. Precision

Precise, mindful execution of the movement and perfect alignment is key to effective Pilates. Moving with precision works the muscles correctly without strain or tension. Correctly aligning your body balances your muscles. Practice giving every aspect of your exercise equal attention, to make each movement more precise and gain more from your workout. Precision also applies to the number of repetitions, your timing, and pace. Bring balance and determination to every aspect of each movement. Memorize the actions and breath patterns of an exercise beforehand, then work on its precise execution. Practice to gain control and skill.

Maintain a long spine as you lengthen the leg away

Reach the leg precisely: Don't allow its weight to drag the spine under

Actively lengthen the heavy, grounded supporting leg

Key points

- **No part of the exercise** should be an afterthought.

- **Imagine your body as an orchestra**: not all instruments take center stage throughout, but all are key to the whole performance. Every part of your body is involved—be aware of what each does throughout.

- **Give equal weight in your mind** to each element of the movement and perform it with care.

5. Breath

Oxygen is vital for correct working of muscles; focusing on the breath ensures they are fully oxygenated during a movement. We breathe in through the nose and out through the mouth, relaxing the jaw and face. Pilates uses "lateral breathing," which channels wide into the body's back and sides so the rib cage expands at the sides as you breathe in, rather than the belly rising forward. Your connection to your center, the abdominals, can then stay strong as you breathe and move. Synchronizing the breath to movement is fundamental in Pilates. We exhale on the effort in Pilates to help engage the deep core muscles effectively.

Key points

- **Often in daily life we breathe shallowly** into our chests. In Pilates, lateral breathing encourages a deeper inhalation, effectively charging your body with fresh oxygen and benefiting your skin, muscles, and blood.

- **Time your breath to the movement.** At first, it seems odd, but with practice it becomes second nature.

- **You should hear your out breath,** like a sigh through soft lips. Don't forget to breathe! If you hold your breath during a movement, you will tense up.

Sigh the breath out through the lips, as if blowing out a candle

As you breathe into the rib cage engage the abdominals so they don't bulge

Feel your breath inflating wide into your back

6. Flowing movements

When practicing Pilates, you should have a silent pulse in your mind, like a metronome or the pulsing of your heart. Perform all exercises synchronized with this pulse and the breath, aiming for continuous, fluid movement. Each exercise is created to flow seamlessly into the next in sequence, with no wasted movement in transition. This ensures a full-body workout that keeps up the heart rate and builds stamina and endurance.

Key points

- **Even in a short workout**, keep your focus and choreograph the sequence of exercises to flow without resting.

- **Pilates appears balletic, strong**, effortless, and not labored, if performed correctly. Aim for the grace and fluidity of a dancer.

Move with an even pace and rhythm

A strong center makes the movement graceful and apparently effortless, despite being hard work

The 6 Key Benefits of Pilates

Pilates exercises combine strengthening with relaxation; they lighten the load on your spine and joints by correcting muscular imbalances due to bad posture or misuse of muscles and also alleviate tension. You'll rediscover your body's natural movement patterns and experience six key benefits.

1. Alignment

Proper alignment balances your skeleton so your muscles are held at their ideal length, without tension. If your body is constantly held in bad alignment, it places a great strain on your muscles, ligaments, and joints, which will reduce your body's ability to react to the force of gravity, resulting in aches and pains and inhibited movement. Pilates gives you an opportunity to learn to correct your misalignments and allow your muscles to work as efficiently as they should.

As you exercise, always strive to correct your alignment because it will directly impact the effectiveness of your workout. Use a mirror where possible to check your alignment and develop your ability to observe how your body moves. Check that your feet are in line with your knees and hips, your shoulders are level, and your waist long. For floor exercises, use the mat as a guide. Work in the center and keep the distances between the sides of the mat and your body equal during the workout.

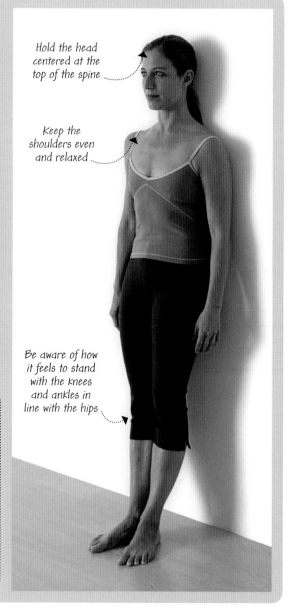

Hold the head centered at the top of the spine

Keep the shoulders even and relaxed

Be aware of how it feels to stand with the knees and ankles in line with the hips

Key benefits

- **The impact of gravity on your spine** and joints will be reduced every day, whether you are moving or at rest.

- **The risk of strain or injury is lessened** with good alignment, particularly with more challenging and dynamic exercises.

- **Improvements in your posture,** how you carry yourself, and how you move every day result from awareness of body alignment.

2. Strength

Pilates is a wonderful body-conditioning program because you don't need any equipment in order to strengthen your body. You can simply use your own body weight to create resistance for your muscles and to tone up—which truly does mean that your workout will be only as effective as the effort you put in to the exercises. Strength begins with a determination to achieve the best. Over time, you will see your muscles gaining tone and looking sculpted; you'll also feel much stronger and more energized.

Pilates strengthens the whole body, targeting each muscle group evenly with a mixture of dynamic and static strength training. No body part is neglected. You also work on all planes of movement—sitting, lying, standing. This means that the muscles are worked from many different directions, producing a uniform and very deep strength and tone, even without using heavy weights.

Key benefits

- **You are less likely to suffer** from muscular and joint aches and pains, or to injure yourself, because your balance and the way you carry yourself will improve.

- **You rev up your metabolism** by building muscle, so that even when not exercising your stronger body burns more calories.

- **Strength leads to greater health:** by committing to a Pilates way of life, you will lower your blood pressure and reduce your cholesterol levels.

- **Pilates builds strength from the inside out,** from your deep core muscles, so that they support your body effectively in movement, and out to your limbs.

- **Reduced tension and strain in the body** results from a strong core, which will also allow your muscles to be free to work with an intensity that will create great results.

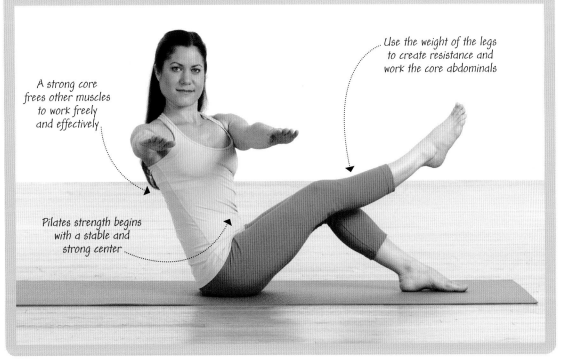

A strong core frees other muscles to work freely and effectively

Use the weight of the legs to create resistance and work the core abdominals

Pilates strength begins with a stable and strong center

3. Flexibility

We all want to achieve a strong body, but there must be a balance between strength and flexibility, and Pilates is the perfect exercise regime to achieve this. Tight muscles hinder your mobility and can lead to tension, aches, and pain. Flexibility is essential for your overall fitness and vitality. It ensures a greater range of movement in your joints, and will in turn mean your joints remain healthy and fare better against normal wear and tear as they age.

Pilates makes most use of dynamic, rather than static, stretching: This involves taking your body into and out of a stretch repeatedly, in a choreographed movement. It warms up the muscles so that they respond more effectively. As you progress through the exercises in this book, you should find your range of movement increasing and your flexibility improving.

Key benefits

- **Your muscles are free from tension** and your movement is unrestricted when you achieve good flexibility.

- **Your posture will improve,** because you will be able to hold your muscles correctly.

- **Better blood circulation** results from improved flexibility, because it helps the muscles align more effectively. Improved circulation also gives you a boost of energy.

- **Joints stay healthy as you age:** They resist wear and tear better if they are flexible and move freely.

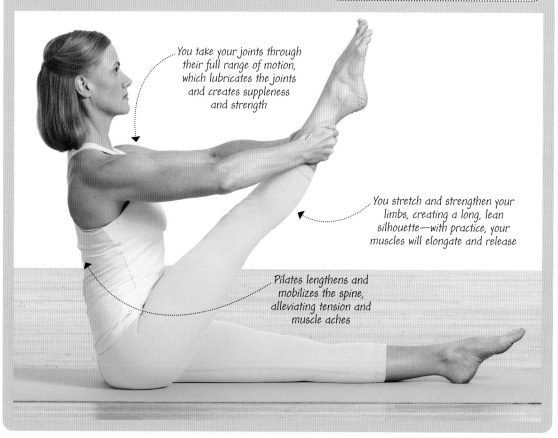

You take your joints through their full range of motion, which lubricates the joints and creates suppleness and strength

You stretch and strengthen your limbs, creating a long, lean silhouette—with practice, your muscles will elongate and release

Pilates lengthens and mobilizes the spine, alleviating tension and muscle aches

4. Shape and tone

For a lot of us, our muscle tone while at rest may be weak. Muscles respond quickly to regular exercise, so after a few weeks of Pilates you should notice visible muscle tone and see your body begin to evolve. The Pilates in this book uses only your body weight and the occasional prop as resistance for shaping your muscles, but it trains every part of your body evenly—front, back, and sides.

For example, during an abdominal exercise, don't think only about engaging your center or belly, but be aware of lengthening your limbs, lifting your buttocks, and connecting your shoulders. If you also combine exercise with proper diet to reduce body fat, you'll notice your muscle tone become even more defined.

Key benefits

- **Develop more muscle definition** through Pilates exercise. Sculpt your waist and shoulders, and tone your abdominals, arms, thighs, and your buttocks.

- **Change your body shape** completely with regular practice of Pilates. With work, you should see a beautifully toned and lengthened body emerge.

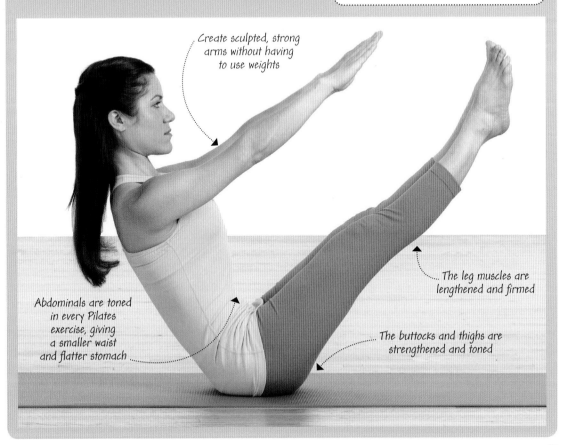

Create sculpted, strong arms without having to use weights

The leg muscles are lengthened and firmed

Abdominals are toned in every Pilates exercise, giving a smaller waist and flatter stomach

The buttocks and thighs are strengthened and toned

5. Endurance

Pilates builds endurance within individual exercises and also within workouts. Focus on improving your concentration to build strength for both—endurance comes first from mental strength and therefore requires determination and persistence. Visualize your success and strength, and stay strong through challenging exercises.

You should practice Pilates sequences without breaks, like a choreographed piece of movement. Initially, you may need to take breaks to perform a linked sequence of exercises. Your muscles will begin to tire after several repetitions, but stay focused and complete the set. Over time, work toward completing a sequence without pausing.

Key benefits

- **Pilates builds stamina**—not only physical, but also mental.

- **Immense strength and tone** in the body is developed in Pilates by using your own body weight.

- **Improved concentration** results from focusing on completing each repetition, exercise, and sequence.

The shoulder muscles work hard to support the weight of the arm through the move

Use your breath and concentration to stay focused and stable even when your muscles start to burn—scan your entire body to release any unnecessary tension

Exercises like Wall: Chair (see p.45) build strength in a static position—sustain the position for a few breaths, using endurance and muscular adjustments throughout to stay strong and controlled

Connect more deeply to your center when you begin to tire

Endurance exercises often challenge large muscle groups, such as the thighs and buttocks

6. Stress Relief

Stress is one of the biggest negative factors of modern life, affecting your physical and mental well-being just as much as disease does. Frequent exercise is one of the best remedies for stress and has many benefits. Pilates focuses on breathing—a deep, mindful pattern of breathing that instantly enhances feelings of calm and release in the body and mind. We also work constantly on posture: a poised and lifted body, free from tension and pain, creates a calm mind.

Release the tension...

Lying on your mat: Before your workout, give in to gravity and consciously release the muscles of the entire body into the floor. Soften the jaw, neck, and shoulders. Feel your worries sink into the mat and leave them there.

The Child's Pose is useful for releasing tension in the back after a challenging exercise. From lying on your front, push your bottom back onto the heels; keep a rounded back and engaged center. Open the knees slightly wider than the hips, to allow the upper body to sink toward the floor. Extend the arms along the mat in front of the head. Inhale to stretch and release the lower back muscles; engage the center more as you exhale.

Key benefits

- **A sense of calm and well-being** is encouraged by the relaxation of tense muscles during Pilates.

- **Pilates releases endorphins**, which naturally cause the body and mind to feel more relaxed and positive.

- **Your sleep will improve** with regular Pilates, which will greatly reduce any fatigue and stress.

- **You will feel energized and invigorated,** because Pilates forces you to focus on the present moment and the movement you are performing, excluding all thought of your everyday preoccupations and stresses.

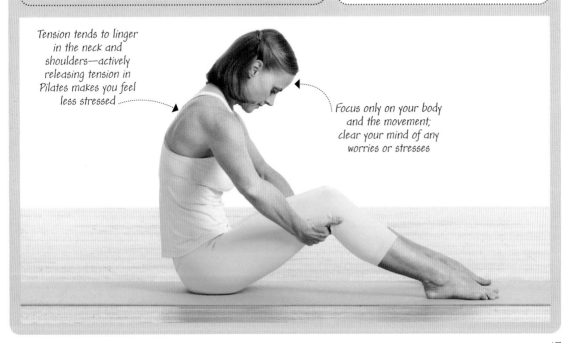

Tension tends to linger in the neck and shoulders—actively releasing tension in Pilates makes you feel less stressed

Focus only on your body and the movement; clear your mind of any worries or stresses

The Science of **Anatomy**

Muscles create movement or stability in the skeleton, holding the bones in correct alignment. Pilates is a unique system that trains the body evenly, restoring balance to muscles and freeing them to perform efficiently. This encourages fluidity of movement and makes you less prone to injury.

Poor posture or overuse makes muscles tight and short, or weak and long. Pilates encourages you to focus on isolating certain body parts and individual or groups of muscles, so you can't use the wrong ones. Understanding more about the musculoskeletal system will enable you to have greater awareness of how to control your body in movement. Imagine your body as an orchestra: like instruments, your muscles should be correctly placed, tuned, and in harmony with each other, and working at the right tempo and volume, with all the bones in the proper placement. Then, you will create the correct movement and work the intended muscles— and soon see them become toned and defined.

In Pilates, muscles work together to create balance, strength, and stamina. You use your own body weight—and props such as hand weights—to create a sculpted and toned body.

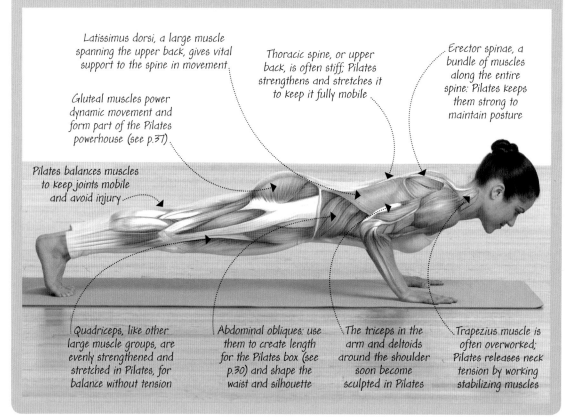

Latissimus dorsi, a large muscle spanning the upper back, gives vital support to the spine in movement.

Gluteal muscles power dynamic movement and form part of the Pilates powerhouse (see p.37).

Thoracic spine, or upper back, is often stiff; Pilates strengthens and stretches it to keep it fully mobile

Erector spinae, a bundle of muscles along the entire spine: Pilates keeps them strong to maintain posture

Pilates balances muscles to keep joints mobile and avoid injury

Quadriceps, like other large muscle groups, are evenly strengthened and stretched in Pilates, for balance without tension

Abdominal obliques: use them to create length for the Pilates box (see p.30) and shape the waist and silhouette

The triceps in the arm and deltoids around the shoulder soon become sculpted in Pilates

Trapezius muscle is often overworked; Pilates releases neck tension by working stabilizing muscles

There are several layers of abdominal muscles and Pilates strengthens each layer. The deepest layer closest to the spine, *transversus abdominis* and pelvic floor, work constantly so need to be strong. More superficial muscles near the skin, such as the obliques and the *rectus abdominis*, tone with movement.

Transversus abdominis and pelvic floor are deep core muscles essential for engaging the scoop (see p.32) and your powerhouse

Rectus abdominis, six-pack abdominals, are vital for stamina and balance: Pilates strengthens them, creating a flat stomach

Humerus and shoulder joint become stronger, moving freely

Femur, or thighbone, gains from strong core control, to support a full range of movement for a healthy hip joint

Cervical spine, the neck, is protected by strong muscles

Adductors, or inner thigh muscles, stabilize the pelvis and thighs and are used in the Pilates stance (see p.35)

Pilates helps the muscles pull your bones into their correct placement

Pectoralis major: these chest muscles are toned in Pilates

Biceps gain strength and tone by using body weight as resistance

The core muscles—the *transversus abdominis*, pelvic floor, and the deep spinal muscles *multifidus*— are strengthened to provide stability, so other muscles are free to move without overworking.

Lumbar spine is vulnerable to pain; Pilates lengthens it, and strengthens muscles supporting it and the back to relieve strain

Sacrum: You feel this part of the spine sink into the mat when lying down for Pilates exercises

Coccyx, or tailbone: Feel this release away from your head, to create length and space in the spine

Ischium, the sit bones: This part of your pelvis releases into the floor in sitting exercises to lengthen your spine

Powerhouse muscles

Use the muscles in your Pilates powerhouse to maintain strength and control in dynamic movements.

- Lift the pelvic floor first (hammock of muscles in the pelvis); glide the sit bones together to engage the muscles, then feel them rising as if moving up floors in an elevator.

- Pull the lower belly in toward the spine to increase engagement and create the "scoop" (see p.32).

- Squeeze your buttocks and inner thighs to start limb movements from a strong, stable core.

The Science of **Alignment**

Pilates trains you to use the deep core muscles of the powerhouse—the abdominals, back, and pelvic floor—to support your posture and bring your skeleton into alignment, so you can move correctly and efficiently.

If the body is constantly held out of good alignment, it puts a great strain on the muscles and joints, compresses the organs, and limits your capacity for deep breathing. This will hinder your body's ability to react against the constant pull of gravity and result in pain and restricted mobility.

Rather than holding your posture with the wrong muscles (such as those around the neck and shoulders, or buttocks) and creating tension where there shouldn't be any, Pilates teaches you how to use your core so your muscles are balanced. It helps you correct your misalignments and imbalances, and achieve the optimal placing of your muscles.

This will allow the shoulders to relax, the neck and head to move freely, and will relieve stress on the lower body. You know good posture when you see it—and we are all inspired by the confidence and strength it radiates.

Side view of ideal alignment: If a plumb line were dropped through the center of the body, it would fall through the middle of the ear and the shoulder, just behind the hip joint and just in front of the ankle joint. Try to imagine this plumb line with your own posture, every day.

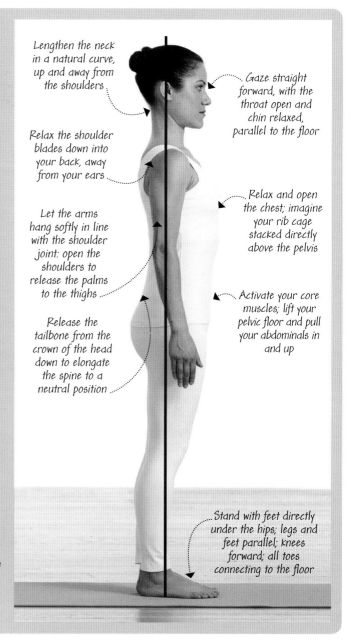

Lengthen the neck in a natural curve, up and away from the shoulders

Gaze straight forward, with the throat open and chin relaxed, parallel to the floor

Relax the shoulder blades down into your back, away from your ears

Relax and open the chest; imagine your rib cage stacked directly above the pelvis

Let the arms hang softly in line with the shoulder joint: open the shoulders to release the palms to the thighs

Activate your core muscles; lift your pelvic floor and pull your abdominals in and up

Release the tailbone from the crown of the head down to elongate the spine to a neutral position

Stand with feet directly under the hips; legs and feet parallel; knees forward; all toes connecting to the floor

Front view of alignment: Imagine you have a space between each vertebra of your spine. Feel these spaces lengthening and the bones lifting up, away from each other, as you grow taller.

Keep the shoulders level and arms released down by your sides

Release the crown of the head to the ceiling; keep your head upright, centered between the shoulders

Lengthen the waist evenly on both sides

Relax your rib cage, so it has enough room to open with your breath

Keep legs straight, but not locked

Hold the hips level and upright with your stabilizing core muscles

Balance your weight evenly, as if it is falling directly through the middle of each foot

Feel yourself floating over the arches of both feet

Science in practice

Good alignment is important to the effectiveness of Pilates exercises; it helps you work the correct muscles and relax parts that shouldn't be working. Proper alignment also lessens the risk of strain or injury.

- Constantly check your alignment: Ensure your feet are in line with the hips, your pelvis is square, and your neck is relaxed and long.

- Use a mirror and mat as a guide for each workout. Work in the center of the mat, keeping the distances between the mat edges and both sides of your body equal as you proceed through the workout.

- Be aware of alignment to improve how you move on a daily basis.

What not to do

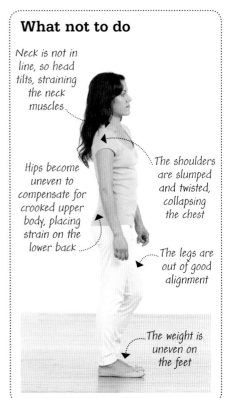

Neck is not in line, so head tilts, straining the neck muscles

Hips become uneven to compensate for crooked upper body, placing strain on the lower back

The shoulders are slumped and twisted, collapsing the chest

The legs are out of good alignment

The weight is uneven on the feet

The Science of **Breathing**

Joe Pilates said, "Above all, learn to breathe correctly." Deep breathing coordinated with movement forms the foundation of all of his exercises. Carry this breathing skill into your daily life and you'll feel energized and calmed, your blood pressure will reduce, and your circulation will improve.

The benefits of efficient, deep breathing, or lateral breathing, cannot be underestimated, yet in daily life we often forget to breathe fully. Joe Pilates saw breathing as a way of cleansing the lungs—he wanted us to "wring the air out of the lungs as water out of a wet cloth." He felt that the exhalation was the most important part of the breath, because a full and long exhalation naturally encourages a deep and wide inhalation, which oxygenates and nourishes the blood and muscles.

Coordinating the breath to the movement is a skill that requires practice and it is what confuses most people when they first begin Pilates. Lateral breathing is an integral part of the Pilates workout: drawing long, deep breaths wide into the sides of the rib cage, followed by a long, full exhalation to deflate the lungs entirely. The exhalation helps to engage the deep abdominal muscles. You can practice lateral breathing while standing up (see below) or lying on the mat.

Correct lateral breathing, wide into the rib cage, exercises the muscles around the rib cage as the lungs expand on the in breath.

Breathing out through the mouth and softening the muscles of the face and jaw allows the neck to relax

Breathing fully into the back allows the ribs to expand out to the sides and the lungs to expand to their fullest capacity

Breathing into the back of the body allows the core abdominal muscles to engage strongly, closing the rib cage and allowing the breath to release

High, shallow breaths into the chest, or "apical" breathing, lift the collarbones, rise the shoulders to the ears, and tense the neck; in lateral breathing, the collarbones and shoulders do not move

Intercostal muscles work to expand the rib cage wide during the in breath; they connect to the obliques, allowing active expulsion of the breath

Breathing in Inhale through the nose, channeling the air fully into the back of the body. Feel under your hands the rib cage expanding sideways with the breath. Soften the shoulders away from the ears.

Breathing out Sigh the breath out through the mouth; relax the jaw. Think of the lungs as bellows, squeezing the air out as the waist muscles wrap around and close the ribs. Feel the rib cage narrow.

Science in practice

The exhalation helps to deeply engage the abdominal muscles.

•Perform movements that need the most powerhouse engagement and effort, such as curling the upper body off the mat, on the out breath.

•Don't let the belly expand with the breath: as you breath in the rib cage expands, then the abdominals contract to expel the out breath.

The Pilates breathing pattern is used to help with the final movement in the Saw (see pp.162–163).

Breathing out as you bend helps the rib cage to close and create a twisting movement

Expelling the breath allows you to engage the abdominals deeply and bend forward farther

Breathing into the back of the body keeps the abdominals engaged as you breathe in and out

The Hundred (see pp.144–145) is the quintessential breathing exercise. You need to coordinate the breath with your movement and breathe efficiently, without tension, as you use the core abdominals.

Sigh the out breath through the mouth to avoid tension in the jaw and neck

Breathing out allows you to scoop the belly; keep it scooped as you breathe in; don't let the belly bulge

Breathe into the back of the body as you deepen your engagement to your center

Essential **Equipment**

For Pilates, all you really need is yourself, but this equipment will help you get the most out of your practice. It is all available online or from sporting goods stores. Wear comfortable, form-fitting clothes without stitching, buttons, or seams that might cause discomfort when you lie on them. Shoes aren't necessary in Pilates: you need to connect your feet into the floor. If you can, work out in front of a mirror, so you can check your alignment.

Magic circle
These are not usually expensive and greatly enhance your workout.

Stretchy band
These are available in various resistances and colors: choose a medium-strength band.

Pilates mat
In Pilates, you need to cushion the spine, so this is thicker than a yoga mat. You could use a thick towel or a blanket, but make sure your spine is comfortable in movement.

Weights
*Choose weights of 2–5lb
(1–2.5kg); heavier ones may
impede the movement. Even a
light weight loads the movement
and you will feel the burn.*

Towel
*Have a towel on hand
—the dynamic exercises
get the blood pumping
and work up a sweat!*

Small cushion
*You may use this under your head when lying on the
mat. Always remove it for exercises such as pelvic curls
(see p.39) or roll overs (see pp.146–147), where you lift
your lower spine, to avoid compressing the neck.*

Water bottle
*It's important to stay hydrated;
if you feel dizzy or light-
headed, stop immediately.*

1
Start Simple

Now that you understand the fundamental principles behind Pilates, you are ready to start putting theory into practice. In this first section, you will be guided through some key techniques and exercises, so that you can create a solid foundation of skills and movements and start developing an awareness of your body's weaknesses and strengths. By the end of this chapter, you will be able to put together what you've learned into an exercise sequence.

Plan Your Program

Joe Pilates said "In 10 sessions you will feel the difference, in 20 you will see the difference, and in 30 you will have a whole new body." Congratulations on committing to Pilates—if you put in the effort, you will soon begin to feel the benefits.

Planning your course

Pilates is a total-body conditioning program; it does not strain the muscles or joints, so the body doesn't need a rest. You can practice every day. (If you have injuries or spinal issues, check with your doctor first.) Take time to understand the key techniques, principles, and exercises. Work through all the warm-up exercises in Key Techniques (see pp.30–39) for your first session. The first week, follow a 15-minute Key Technique sequence each day—try to perfect each technique and become familiar with the muscular engagement. Then, begin the Start Simple program. Aim to apply the six Pilates principles every time you practice.

Start Simple Exercise Program

Use this program to set yourself goals and assess your progress over the next six weeks. (Sequence summaries are on pp.80–85.) Each week, follow the sequences exactly and focus on one area. As the weeks pass, more will be added until, by the end of the course, you should feel comfortable concentrating on multiple aspects of your movement. Then you could substitute other exercises with the same level of proficiency, as long as they train the same body area, for a balanced workout. Pilates is all about detail. Be your own coach: check every movement. If you find it easy, you may not be performing it attentively.

Week 1: Focus on Alignment

Baseline: Take photos of yourself standing— front, side, and back—and draw plumb lines on the images, as on pp.20–21.

- **Day 1:** 15-minute sequence, check scoop
- **Day 2:** 15-minute sequence, check lengthening
- **Day 3:** 15-minute sequence, check precision
- **Day 4:** 15-minute sequence, check stability
- **Day 5:** 15-minute sequence, check C-curve

Goal: Take new photos after six weeks to see how much closer you are to the ideal alignment.

Week 2: Focus on Control

Baseline: Perform the Roll Back (see pp.56–57). Are you shaking, tensing, misaligned, or moving jerkily? Is your Pilates box square?

- **Day 1:** 15-minute sequence, check centering, alignment
- **Day 2:** 30-minute sequence, check concentration, precision
- **Day 3:** 15-minute sequence, check precision, breathing
- **Day 4:** 30-minute sequence, check flowing movement, stability
- **Day 5:** 15-minute sequence, check lengthening, breathing

Goal: Do the exercise with control, precision, and fluidity, remembering

to breathe, scoop, and lengthen.

Week 3: Focus on Centering

Baseline: Perform the Centering exercise (see p.40). Is the spine supported and strong as you move? Is the back arched?
• **Day 1:** 15-minute sequence, check Pilates box, alignment, flowing movement
• **Day 2:** 30-minute sequence, check stability, precision, lengthening
• **Day 3:** 45-minute sequence, check precision, control, breathing
• **Day 4:** 30-minute sequence, check control, alignment
• **Day 5:** 15-minute sequence, check alignment, scoop
Goal: Perform the exercise with no spinal movement as you lengthen the limbs away, smoothly and with control.

Week 4: Focus on Flexibility

Baseline: Perform Wall: Roll Down (see pp.42–43). Does your spine feel mobile and fluid or stiff and inflexible?
• **Day 1:** 15-minute sequence, check precision, control, alignment
• **Day 2:** 30-minute sequence, check breathing, scoop, stability
• **Day 3:** 45-minute sequence, check scoop, powerhouse, coordination
• **Day 4:** 30-minute sequence, check control, concentration
• **Day 5:** 15-minute sequence, check alignment, flowing movement
Goal: Move fluidly, bone by bone, and achieve even sequential movement through each part of the spine.

Week 5: Focus on Strength

Baseline: Perform Wall: Chair (see p.45), Hundred Preparation (see pp.54–55), and Roll Up, pp.58–59) without a break. On a scale of 1–10, how hard is each exercise and sequence?
• **Day 1:** 15-minute sequence, check centering, control, coordination
• **Day 2:** 45-minute sequence, check scoop, alignment, concentration
• **Day 3:** 15-minute sequence, check flowing movement, alignment, coordination
• **Day 4:** 30-minute sequence, check control, precision, powerhouse
• **Day 5:** 45-minute sequence, check flowing movement, breathing
Goal: Performing the sequence should feel easier.

Week 6: Focus on Flowing Movement

Baseline: Perform Single Leg Stretch 1 (see p.64). Are you moving fluidly or jerkily? Can you link both leg movements smoothly?
•**Day 1:** 30-minute sequence, check centering, breathing, coordination
•**Day 2:** 45-minute sequence, check stability, control, Pilates box
•**Day 3:** 15-minute sequence, check alignment, precision, coordination
•**Day 4:** 30-minute sequence, check precision, centering, breathing
•**Day 5:** 45-minute sequence, check control, powerhouse, concentration
Goal: Do the exercise swiftly, changing from side to side without wobbling or stopping.

There is a lot to take on board when you start Pilates, but as you gain confidence and skill, your practice will improve. Pilates will lift your spirits and give you a new body.

Your breathing, stamina, and strength will improve; you'll move more gracefully and see muscle definition and a sculpted shape emerging. Enjoy the next six weeks!

Key Techniques to Practice

In Pilates, there are a few fundamental positions you need to master to ensure your workout is safe and effective. Practice these positions until you feel them confidently and correctly in your body, and revisit them regularly as you advance through the levels.

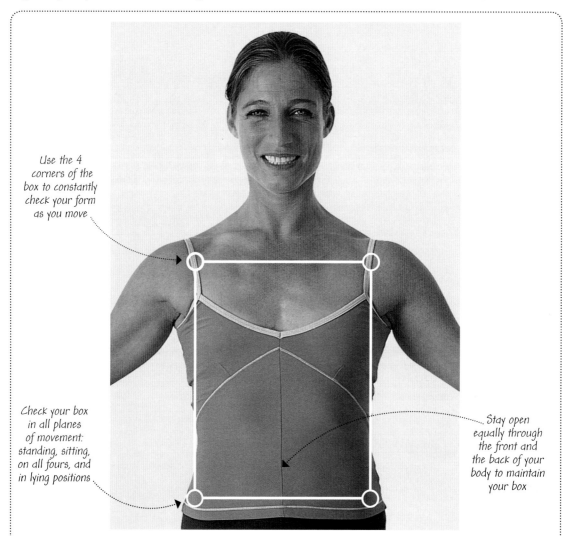

Use the 4 corners of the box to constantly check your form as you move

Check your box in all planes of movement: standing, sitting, on all fours, and in lying positions

Stay open equally through the front and the back of your body to maintain your box

The Pilates box

This box is your reference for checking your alignment, making sure your muscles are balanced, and reminding you to work symmetrically and safely. Check that your box remains square while you move. Be aware of whether you're twisted or shortening on one side. Train yourself to notice differences in length on either side of your body.

Visualize a triangle of your hip bones and pubic bone, level and parallel with the floor

Feel the natural curves of your spine releasing into the mat, and your muscles balanced and ready for action

Neutral spine

Arching places stress on the lower back muscles

Arching the back

Tucking under will cause you to lose the natural curve of your lower spine

Tucking under

The neutral spine

Neutral spine encourages length in the spine, in its natural curve. In neutral, muscles are switched off, perfectly balanced, and your body primed for movement. As you lie flat on the floor, roll through the pelvis, tilting forward and back. Gradually decrease the movement and come to a point where you're neither arched nor tucking. This is neutral.

Tummy has protruded

Bad scoop

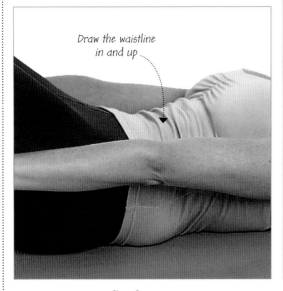

Draw the waistline in and up

Good scoop

Standing scoop

The scoop

The scoop should look and feel as if you're hollowing your abdominals up and in. The abdominals should move deep toward the spine, pinning your navel like a mattress button, without affecting the natural curve of your spine. It should feel as if you're pulling in a corset, tightly drawing the waist in and up, and engaging the lower abdominals.

No part of the body is shortened or hunched

Imagine someone is pulling your leg up toward the ceiling

Lengthening

In Pilates, we continually aim to lengthen our body using our muscles. To elongate the waist, lift the ribs away from the hips and create space between each vertebra of the spine, growing taller and longer throughout the movement. You will often see directions to "lift," "lengthen," and "reach." Every movement is consciously sustaining a long spine and limbs, so you are aware of your posture and every part of your body, even if it's not moving. After a good Pilates session, you should feel taller, and you may actually be taller!

Tip The core, also called the "center," refers to a layer of muscles that encircle the spine and pelvis. They are stabilizing muscles, since they create strength and support the spine, but they do not control the dynamic movement of the spine or limbs. The core, along with mobilizing muscles, forms the powerhouse (see p.37). Also see Science of Anatomy on p.18.

Deepen the abdominals as much as you can while staying relaxed in the rest of the body

Leg lengthens away as the buttocks and spine stay lifted

Imagine the torso is anchored as you move the limbs freely

Stabilizing

In Pilates, we need to keep the torso stable as we move. This means that no unwanted movement should occur in the body while we move our limbs. To do this, we need to engage our core muscles: the pelvic floor, deep abdominals, and spinal muscles. This supports and stabilizes the spine, and enables the limbs to move freely without tension.

Warm-up Exercises

Before each Pilates workout, you must warm up your body. Take a few minutes to practice one, or all, of these exercises to mobilize the spine, focus on your breathing, and relax your muscles in preparation for movement. The seated C-curve (see p.36) and Pilates stance (see opposite) are positions that you need to create in many exercises shown in this book. Learn to engage your powerhouse (see p.37) correctly to move with energy, stability, strength, and control. Remember to practice your key techniques as you perform these exercises.

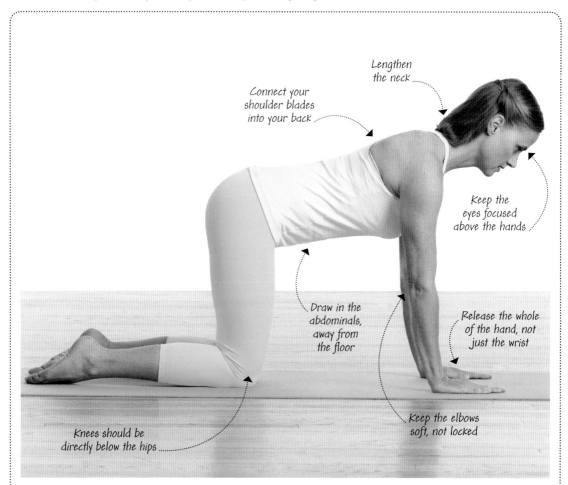

Lengthen the neck

Connect your shoulder blades into your back

Keep the eyes focused above the hands

Draw in the abdominals, away from the floor

Release the whole of the hand, not just the wrist

Knees should be directly below the hips

Keep the elbows soft, not locked

The table top

This is an exercise in concentration and alignment, requiring strength and balance. Align yourself on all fours, hands beneath the shoulders and knees beneath the hips. Your spine is in neutral (see p.31). On an out breath, draw your pelvic floor and lower belly up and in. Breathe in to hold this position. As you breathe out, gently release. Repeat this 5 times.

Relax the shoulders

Feel open across the chest

Engage your buttock muscles and rotate the thighbones to open the toes apart

Squeeze the legs from the inner thighs and the buttocks

Feet in parallel

Feet in Pilates stance

The Pilates stance

You'll find this position in many Pilates exercises, working the powerhouse (see p.37), buttock muscles, and inner thighs. Stand upright, spine in neutral (see p.31), arms down by your sides. Begin with the feet in parallel, toes and heels together. As you breathe out, open the feet. Keep the weight even through all 10 toes. Repeat this 5 times.

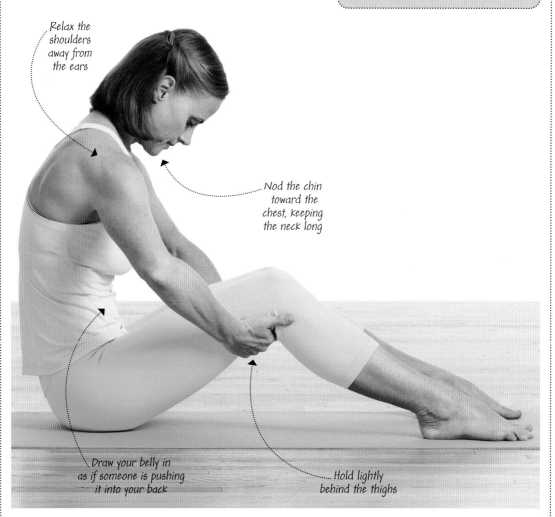

Careful! Never slump the spine forward. It should feel active and lifted in this position. Relax the shoulders, elbows wide.

Relax the shoulders away from the ears

Nod the chin toward the chest, keeping the neck long

Draw your belly in as if someone is pushing it into your back

Hold lightly behind the thighs

The seated C-curve

The C-curve requires the ability to scoop your abdominals (see p.32) without affecting the position of the spine, mobilizing the spine with control. Sit tall, with knees bent and legs hip-width apart. Place your hands behind your thighs. Breathe deeply into the back of your body. As you breathe out, scoop the abdominals, lifting the ribcage away from the hips, and curl your tailbone underneath to roll the spine into a C-shape. Your shoulders are in line with your hips. Repeat this 5 times.

Relax the shoulders

Keep one hand on your belly and the other on your lower back

Feel the breath into the belly, expanding into your hand

Inhale

Keep the waist long

Draw the tummy away from your hand toward your spine

Wrap the buttock muscles around

Draw the powerhouse up and in, tightening the waist and closing the rib cage

Exhale

The powerhouse

The powerhouse (see p.10), a term coined by Joe Pilates, refers to the core muscles (see p.19), plus strong mobilizing muscles, such as the six-pack abdominals, inner thighs, and buttocks. He also called it your "girdle of strength," a corset of muscles supporting the torso, stabilizing the body, and allowing power for movement. Here we learn to recruit the powerhouse, engaging the muscles appropriately and slowly, like a dimmer switch. Repeat 8 times. Stay soft and still in the spine as you engage the muscles.

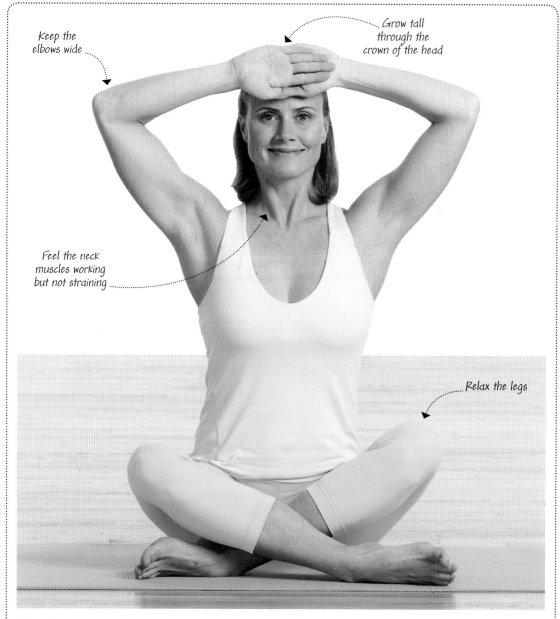

Keep the elbows wide

Grow tall through the crown of the head

Feel the neck muscles working but not straining

Relax the legs

Neck presses

This is a posture check that encourages length in your spine and relaxes the neck. Sit cross-legged on your mat, evenly on both sit bones. Place the back of one hand on your forehead, with your other hand placed on top of it. Lengthen the crown of your head up toward the ceiling as you press the head into the hands, resisting the movement with your neck muscles. Don't allow the neck to move backward. Hold for 2 breaths. Repeat 5 times.

38

Relax the bottom before you begin, and make sure the hips are relaxed

Press the arms into the ground to support your weight

Feel heavy through the feet

Reach the thighs away as you lift

Draw the belly in

Curl the tailbone underneath you

Pelvic curls

Focus on spinal alignment and the sequential mobility of the spine, moving evenly, bone by bone, like a wheel. Lie on your back with your feet flat on the floor, hip-width apart. Relax the head. Breathe in to prepare. As you breathe out, connect to your powerhouse and curl the tailbone under, releasing the lower spine into the mat. Then, lift the buttocks to peel the spine off the floor slightly. Breathe in as you lower, slowly. Repeat 5 times.

Centering

Strengthen Core • **Practice** Control

This is a great way to strengthen your core (the muscles that protect your lower back, abdominals, and pelvic floor). Revisit it regularly to reinforce the feeling in your body and strengthen the connection to your powerhouse (see p.37).

1 Lie on your back with knees bent and feet flat on the floor. Release your body onto the floor with your breath. Relax the hips. Relax the shoulders and connect to your abdominals. Breathe in to prepare.

Spine in neutral is perfectly balanced, belly slightly pulled in and scooped

Knees hip-width apart, bent up to the ceiling

Weight evenly spread through the feet

Long and straight arm, reaching directly in line with the shoulder

Keep the foot softly pointed

2 Breathe out, and lengthen one arm back, simultaneously stretching the opposite leg forward, in line with the body. Keep the spine long and still. Float the arm and leg back as you breathe in. Alternate sides. Repeat up to 8 times on each side.

More of a challenge

Stretch both arms and legs together. Hold your spine stable by scooping your belly deeply to anchor the torso. Keep your arms in line with the ears.

Careful! Don't allow your back to arch as you stretch.

Keep your legs connected

Softly point the feet as you reach the legs away

Neck Peels

Strengthen Stomach • **Practice** Precision

This tones the abdominal muscles, while keeping the neck free from strain. Allow the weight of your head to be carried entirely by your arms and the band, not by the neck.

1 Lie centrally on top of a band or towel, placed underneath your tailbone and the entire length of the spine, with your feet flat on the floor. Soften the ribs toward the hips.

Keep knees hip-width apart

Hold onto the band with both hands, with some tension in the band

Don't arch your back

Be careful not to tuck the pelvis under

2 Breathe out, scoop your abdominals by drawing your waistline in and up, and gently peel the head and shoulder blades off the mat, feeling the head heavy on the band, and no strain in the neck. Breathe in at the top of the curl, and breathe out to release down slowly. Repeat 5 times.

Keep elbows soft and wide

Imagine that your neck is completely light and free from tension

Press evenly into the feet

Wall: Roll Down

Strengthen Stomach • **Practice** Flowing Movement

Roll downs challenge your abdominals by working against gravity to rebuild the spine sequentially. Resist the curl forward by constantly lifting your belly.

1 Stand against the wall with your feet slightly away from the wall, in Pilates stance. Your spine should be neutral, neither arched nor tucked under.

Why? We use the belly muscles to support and mobilize the spine. It's important to learn how to recruit them correctly, working against gravity.

Keep your head aligned to the top of the spine

If your head doesn't naturally meet the wall, don't force it

Open the shoulders back

Arms relaxed toward the floor

Legs rotated in Pilates stance, with heels together and feet slightly apart

Take care...

If you feel a strain in your neck or shoulders, build the movement up slowly until you have released all tension. Learn to let go of your arms and neck completely.

Don't let your tailbone move up the wall. Be careful not to hinge at the hips. Keep the pelvis upright by scooping the abdominals.

Don't let your abdominals collapse forward. Feel the movement coming from your center, peeling the spine off the wall and then replacing it smoothly.

2 As you breathe out, scoop the belly, nod the nose down, and peel the spine from the wall: first the head, then the shoulders.

Imagine Peel the top of your spine away from the wall like a drooping flower, while the rest stays anchored and lifted.

Remember "Scoop your belly" means to hollow your abdominals up and in.

3 Roll the spine as far as you can without allowing the tailbone to rise up. Keep the pelvis upright. Breathe in. Then breathe out and re-stack the spine to standing, bone by bone. Repeat up to 10 times.

Imagine Draw the belly in really deeply, as if you're hanging over a clothesline.

The belly is lifted and tailbone is heavy against the wall

Arms hang loose by your sides

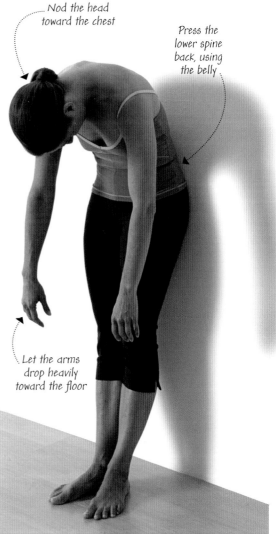

Nod the head toward the chest

Press the lower spine back, using the belly

Let the arms drop heavily toward the floor

Wall: Stand

Strengthen Core • **Practice** Centering and Breathing

This is a fantastic posture check that you can do anywhere,
any time: at home, at work, or at play. It's a great way
to connect to your body.

Keep your collarbones wide and shoulders soft and open

Relax arms down by your sides

Lift up into your center

Wrap the leg muscles around in Pilates stance

Keep toes apart, spread evenly on the floor

Stand at the wall, with your feet slightly away and your legs in Pilates stance. Lean back, spine in neutral and head heavy into the wall. Scan your body: check your neck is released, your ribs are connected to your hips, and your lower back is long. Breathe wide and full into your back, and ensure you are connected to your center. Repeat for as long as you need to relax your spine and center your body.

Wall: Chair

Strengthen Arms and Legs • **Practice** Control

This move requires focus and strength, and uses weights to
tone the arms. You'll feel your thighs burning! Avoid this
exercise if you have knee problems.

Keep your
collarbones
wide, shoulders
released
against the wall

Hands in line with the
arms and holding the
weights firmly

Place the
feet in
parallel

Be careful not to
tense the neck: stay
soft and long

Keep the
wrists in good
alignment with
the arms

Bend the
knees at 90°

1 Stand tall, with your feet hip-width
apart. Place your feet slightly farther
away from the wall than in Wall: Stand
(see opposite). Hold the hand weights and
relax your arms by your sides.

2 Breathe in. As you breathe out, slide
your spine down the wall to "sit," with
your knees directly over the ankles. Float
the arms up to shoulder height, palms down.
Hold for 5 breaths. Repeat, increasing the
number of breaths each time, working up
to 10. Breathe out as you slide back up,
lowering the arms as you do so.

Wall: Circles

Strengthen Shoulders • **Practice** Flowing Movement

Here we learn to move the arms freely with control, while
keeping the center strong. You can also do this
with hand weights for arm toning.

1 Stand against the wall, feet
slightly away from the wall,
shoulders wide. Float your arms
forward and up to shoulder
height. Scoop the belly to support
the lower back, feeling it releasing
toward the wall, spine in neutral.

Imagine As you stand, imagine
your neck lengthening away from
the rest of the spine, lifting the
crown of the head up to the ceiling.

Reach the hands out
long and soft,
in line with
the shoulders

Keep the rib cage
connected into the
body and heavy
against the wall

Legs in Pilates
stance, squeezing
from the inner thighs
and buttocks

Open the feet, toes
spread evenly

Take care...

If your neck feels tense, imagine
the movement coming from the
center of the shoulder blades, floating
the arms from your rib cage rather
than from the neck.

Don't let your spine arch or tuck
under—keep it in neutral. Keep the
belly pulled in slightly and scooped.

Don't let your arms move at
a different pace. Concentrate and
control the movement, coordinating
the movement of each arm in time
with the other.

2 Open the arms out to the sides, keeping them in your peripheral vision. Keep the shoulders integrated into your body. Draw the abdominals deeper up and in.

Careful! Don't open your arms too wide or you will arch your back.

3 Float the arms down toward the hips once more. Keep the neck reaching up toward the ceiling, with your spine long and relaxed. Lower the arms to just in front of the hips. Repeat the circle 3 times in each direction, breathing naturally.

Keep the arms in your sight, reaching away

Draw the belly deeply into the spine

Rotate and squeeze the legs together

Keep the shoulders soft, away from the ears

Keep the hand in line with the rest of the arm

Squeeze the backs of the thighs together

Biceps: Front Curls

Strengthen Arms • **Practice** Precision

These exercises are great for toning arms. Connect to your powerhouse and make this an all-body exercise. Imagine you're working under water to offer more resistance to your muscles.

Connect the shoulders into the body

Bring weights toward you

Reach the forearms out in front of the shoulders, palms up

Bend the elbows at 90°

Keep the spine long and don't arch it

Belly lifted in and up

Wrap the legs together in Pilates stance, squeezing the buttocks and inner thighs

Spread the toes evenly

1 Stand tall, in Pilates stance, holding a weight in each hand. Connect strongly from your heels up to the inner thighs and buttocks. Scoop the belly. Float the arms forward to shoulder height, palms facing up. Keep the elbows unlocked.

2 Bend both arms in toward you, keeping the elbows level. Breathe in to bend the arms in, and out to lengthen them away. Repeat 5 times, working up to 10.

Careful! Don't tense the neck or lean back. Keep the shoulders away from the ears.

Biceps: Side Curls

Strengthen Arms • **Practice** Centering

Holding the arms out to the sides focuses on slightly different muscles. Here we tone the deltoids (shoulder muscles) as well as the biceps. Stay strongly connected to your center throughout.

Palm open to the ceiling, fingers closed over the weight

Rib cage closed into the body, waist long

Inner thighs squeezing in Pilates stance

Keep the upper arm level as you fold the forearm in

Connect the muscles around the rib cage and waist to keep your center strong

Feel the inner thighs wrapping toward each other

Place the feet evenly down into the ground

1 Float your arms out to the sides, in your peripheral vision, with your palms facing up. Keep your shoulders soft, ribs connected into the torso, belly deeply scooped.

Imagine As you move, imagine the crown of your head being lifted to the ceiling.

2 Curl the arms up, bending the elbows to about 90°. Relax the shoulders and keep the elbows level. Scoop in the belly deeply. Repeat 5 times, building up to 10. Breathe in to bend the arms in, and out to extend them away.

Boxing

Strengthen Arms • **Practice** Control

This tones and sculpts the arms and shoulders and requires
a lot of core strength. Be strict with yourself, and really control
your movements, and you'll see results in no time.

1 Stand tall, with your feet
hip-width apart and parallel.
Bend the knees over the toes,
scoop the belly, and hinge
forward, keeping the back long.
Bend your arms upward to bring
the hands to the shoulders. Keep
your elbows into your waist and
feel your shoulder blades snug into
your back. Breathe in to prepare.

Remember Stay soft and long
in the neck, and keep the weight
even on both feet.

Keep the back
long belly deeply
drawn in

Feel the
buttocks and
backs of the
thighs working

Make sure your
hands are in line
with the arms

Keep feet in
parallel, evenly
grounded

Keep the
belly lifted
and in

Keep your
face parallel
with the floor,
eyes focused
downward

Reach the
arm in
line with
your ears

2 As you breathe out, reach the
right arm forward and the left
arm back, pressing the fists away.
Breathe in to bring them back to
center. Repeat 3 sets. Roll the
spine down and allow the arms to
release toward the floor. Breathe
out and roll the spine up, bone by
bone, back to standing.

Careful! Try not to let your arms
drop: they should reach in line with
the shoulders. Keep the belly lifted
and the shoulder blades connected
into the back.

Standing Side Bends

Strengthen Waist • **Practice** Flowing Movement

This is a wonderful way to tone the oblique muscles in the waist, as well as the shoulders. Move smoothly, with control, and you'll soon see the results.

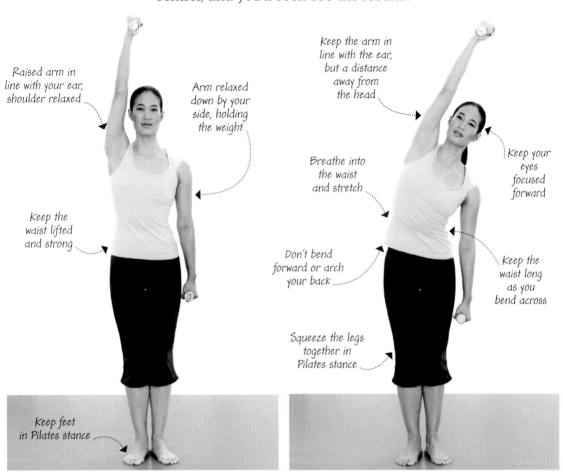

Raised arm in line with your ear, shoulder relaxed

Arm relaxed down by your side, holding the weight

Keep the arm in line with the ear, but a distance away from the head

Breathe into the waist and stretch

Keep your eyes focused forward

Keep the waist lifted and strong

Don't bend forward or arch your back

Keep the waist long as you bend across

Squeeze the legs together in Pilates stance

Keep feet in Pilates stance

1 Stand in Pilates stance. Breathe in to lengthen the right arm up above you, in line with your ear. Draw the belly in and relax the neck. Keep the shoulder soft and away from the ear. Lift the crown of your head toward the ceiling. Plant your feet down into the ground.

2 Breathe out, reach the right arm up, and across to the left. Relax the left arm down by your side. Breathe in, feeling a stretch in the right side. Breathe out, return to center, and lower the right arm. Repeat on the other side. Perform 6 repetitions.

Chest Expansion

Strengthen Arms and Upper Back • **Practice** Breathing

This is a great way to open the chest and work the muscles of the upper back, between the shoulder blades. Try to do this every day, to counteract a slumping posture.

1 Stand tall in Pilates stance, strongly engaging the inner thighs and buttocks. Float both arms in front of the body, palms down, shoulders relaxed.

Imagine As you exercise, imagine the crown of your head and neck extending to the ceiling. Direct your eyes down toward the floor, nodding the chin gently toward the chest.

Shoulders relaxed and down

Keep the fingers long and energized

Take care...

Don't arch your back. Keep your spine lengthened and stable as you move the arms. When you press the arms behind, draw deeper into your center to make sure you resist the spine arching.

Try not to rock on your feet. Keep your weight evenly grounded through the feet as you move the arms. Stay connected with the legs and spread the weight through all 10 toes and your heels.

The body shouldn't twist with the head. Make sure this is a movement just in the neck, free from the torso.

Buttocks and inner thighs engaged

Feet open in Pilates stance

2 Breathe in, and press your arms back, feeling the triceps activate as you reach the arms behind you. Feel the shoulder blades drawing inward.

Careful! Avoid arching the back. Keep your waist long and belly lifted.

3 Look over the right shoulder, then the left. Return to center. Breathe out to glide the arms back to the front of the body. Repeat, alternating your gaze, turning your head from left to right, then right to left. Repeat each set 3 times, trying to open the chest more every time.

Feel the triceps in the upper arms working to bring the arms behind you

Reach the fingertips long

Legs are rotated and squeezing together

Keep the arms long and straight

Squeeze the buttocks

Press the feet evenly into the floor

Hundred Preparation

Strengthen Stomach • **Practice** Breathing

This tough exercise may not become your favorite, but it
is very effective. This is a classic breathing exercise
in Pilates, and targets the deep abdominals.

1 Sit tall, feet hip-width apart.
Hold behind your thighs lightly.
Draw the abdominals in and up.
Breathe in. As you breathe out,
curl the tailbone under, and begin
to roll down onto the mat.

Why? Breathing fully and moving
on the out breath helps to engage
the abdominals strongly. Breathing
into the back of the rib cage is the
only way to perform this exercise
smoothly and correctly.

Keep your eyes
focused forward

Don't collapse
the chest

Elbows wide
and soft

Legs hip-width
apart and parallel

Take care...

Don't let your feet lift. Keep the
feet heavy and grounded into the
floor, and allow this to help you
connect to your abdominals.

Your body shouldn't move as the
arms pump freely. Keep your scoop
strong and make sure the spine
doesn't move.

Try not to tilt your head back.
Keep the eyes focused in toward your
navel and the neck long.

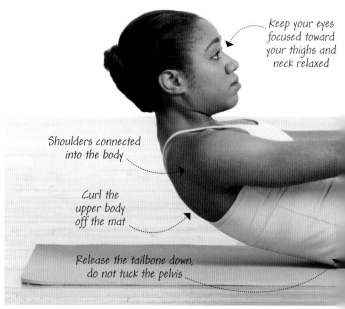

Keep your eyes
focused toward
your thighs and
neck relaxed

Shoulders connected
into the body

Curl the
upper body
off the mat

Release the tailbone down,
do not tuck the pelvis

Lengthen your head at the end of your spine

Arms open and relaxed

2 Curl down with control, keeping the eyes focused forward, not up. Engage your abdominals to release the lower spine toward the mat. Keep the upper body curled off the mat and the chest open.

Knees straight up toward the ceiling

Keep your feet heavy into the floor

3 Release the arms forward. Breathe in and pump the arms for 5 counts, then breathe out and pump for 5 counts. Continue pumping until you reach 50. Breathe out and roll back up to sitting.

Tip Pump the arms down toward the floor and up toward the knees, as if you are bobbing a ball underneath. Your shoulders should move freely in the joints and the arms should move as one unbroken unit from shoulder to fingertip. Don't allow the hands to flop or bend the wrists or elbows.

Reach the arms long, out of the shoulder joints

Keep the feet heavy into the mat

Pump the arms up and down in short, dynamic movements

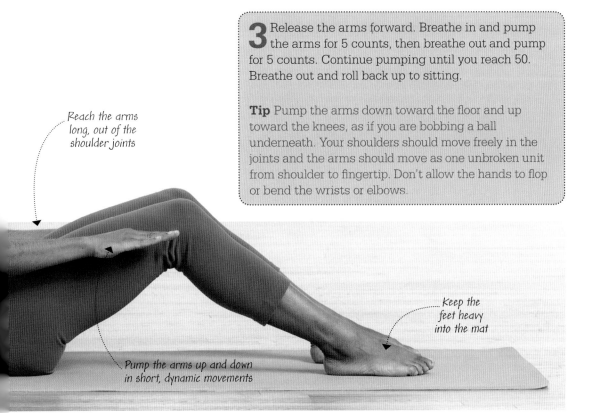

Roll Back

Strengthen Stomach • **Practice** Control

This exercise requires a deep connection to your powerhouse to help you move. Check this connection throughout the exercise so you don't let it slip. It's great practice for more advanced work.

Connect the shoulders into your back

Keep your spine straight and strong

Keep your elbows wide

1 Sit tall, with the feet grounded and hip-width apart. Place your hands lightly under your thighs. Scoop your belly and lengthen your waist. Breathe in to prepare.

Imagine To keep your waist long, imagine you have elastic bands connecting your ribs down toward your hips. Try to keep the bands taut; don't allow them to expand and lose the connection.

Keep the feet heavy

Keep elbows soft and wide

Lift crown of the head to the ceiling

Draw your shoulders into the body

Take care...

Don't hinge from the hip. The movement should be a rolling C-curve from the tailbone, and not straight from the upper back.

Avoid arching the back and allowing the ribs to pop forward. Keep the abdominals strong.

Don't look up to the ceiling. Keep the neck long and eyes focused toward your center.

2 Breathe out, deepen your abdominals, and curl the tailbone underneath to roll your lower back toward the mat. Nod the chin to the chest to finish the C-curve of the spine.

Use the belly to support the lower back

Keep the knees hip-width apart and pointed at the ceiling

Connect the shoulders into the body

Press forward through the lower legs

3 Scoop more and release the mid-back into the mat. Hold this position for 3 breaths. As you breathe out each time, pull your belly in more. Keep the deep engagement to roll the spine back up to the sitting position, on an out breath. Repeat 3 times.

Careful! Keep the waist long on both sides. Think about your box and try not to collapse on one side.

Keep your legs hip-width apart

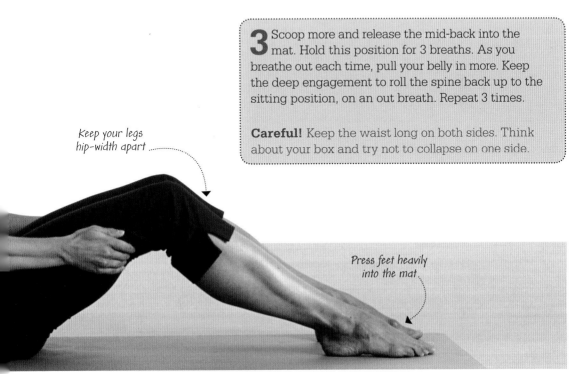

Press feet heavily into the mat

Roll Up

Strengthen Stomach • **Practice** Control and Breathing

This wonderful exercise works on your strength, flexibility, and control. We move the spine sequentially, rolling each part evenly like a wheel, using the abdominals strongly.

1 Lie flat on the mat and lengthen your arms overhead, in line with your ears. Connect the ribs down. Squeeze your inner thighs and flex your feet.

Remember All the principles of Pilates are illustrated in this exercise, and your body will feel the effects if you take the time to perfect the movement.

Reach arms in line with the ears

Open palms to the ceiling

Relax the rib cage down

2 Breathe in; float the arms above the shoulders. Nod the chin toward the chest; look down toward your center. Scoop the belly deeply and flex the feet.

Reach your arms straight above the shoulders

Lengthen the neck to look forward

Press out through the heels

3 Breathe out and curl the upper body off the mat, lifting the ribs and deepening the abdominals. Press the arms forward and toward the toes.

Imagine Think of your spine as a string of pearls: you're picking the pearls up one by one, then smoothly laying them down again.

Keep the arms long and straight

Keep the crown of the head lifted

Reach toes to the ceiling

Connect shoulders into the body

4 Breathe in; draw the belly in as you roll forward over your legs, reaching the arms to your toes. Breathe out to roll the spine back down to the mat, bone by bone. As your shoulders meet the mat, reach the arms back behind you. Repeat the exercise 5 times.

Connect the shoulders into the body by drawing the shoulder blades into the back

Keep the waist lifted and belly scooped

Palms face down to the floor

Curl tailbone underneath in a C-curve

Make it easier

If you can't control the movement, bend the knees slightly and place your hands under your thighs to help you support yourself while you build strength. Move slowly through each part of the spine.

Keep the knees soft

Arms reach behind the thighs

Leg Circles

Strengthen Thighs and Buttocks
Practice Concentration and Precision

It takes a lot of control to ensure there is no unwanted
movement in the body. Use your powerhouse (see p.37) in this
exercise to anchor the torso while the legs move.

1 Lying on the mat, align yourself centrally on your
back, with one leg bent and the other extended up
in the air, in line with the hip. Scoop the belly. Relax
the spine into neutral.

Remember The purpose of this exercise is to control
your movement, so keep your torso stable and use your
abdominals for control.

Point the
foot softly

Leg rotated
in Pilates
stance

Keep the
waist long

Side view

Draw the
belly in
and up

Keep the supporting
leg steady

Press the foot
into the floor

2 Connect to your center and sweep the extended leg across the body, using the inner thigh muscles. Aim the big toe toward your opposite shoulder.

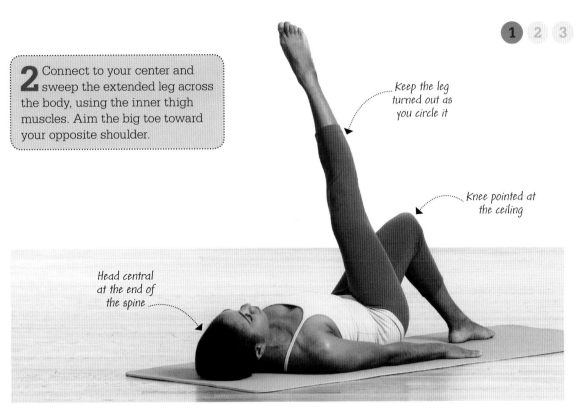

Keep the leg turned out as you circle it

Knee pointed at the ceiling

Head central at the end of the spine

3 Circle the leg down and around, and back up to center. Breathe in for the first half of the circle, out for the second. Repeat 8 times in each direction. Make the circles precise and even.

Why? Leg circles encourage freedom of movement without affecting a strong core. In Pilates, isolating certain parts—like the thighs and buttocks here—ensures your muscles are balanced and no tension is introduced anywhere.

Foot lengthens away

Keep the leg turned out

Feel anchored through the rib cage

Supporting foot heavy and grounded

Relax arms and neck

Rolling Like a Ball 1

Strengthen Stomach • **Practice** Flowing Movement

This playful exercise is surprisingly challenging for your core. Work hard to maintain your C-curve for a smooth and flowing movement. Practice it swiftly, for flow, and slowly, to develop your concentration and control.

1 Sit tall on your mat. Hold the backs of the thighs lightly. Use your abdominals to float your legs up, shins parallel with the floor, tipping back off your sit bones. Curl into a C-curve (see p.36) and balance for a moment to prepare.

Imagine Think of a ball encircling your body, so when you roll back, you roll smoothly and continuously.

Knees hip-width apart

Keep feet together

Keep elbows soft and open

Pull your abdominals in and curl your tailbone under

Feet reach to the ceiling

Keep eyes focused on the belly throughout the roll

Hands behind the thighs

Waist long on both sides

2 Breathe in, and roll back smoothly. As you roll to your shoulder blades, maintain your body shape and lengthen your tailbone to the ceiling. Stay long in the neck and relaxed in the shoulders, keeping the belly strong to make sure your spine doesn't straighten.

Careful! Don't roll too far. Roll only as far as the shoulders: the head should not touch the floor.

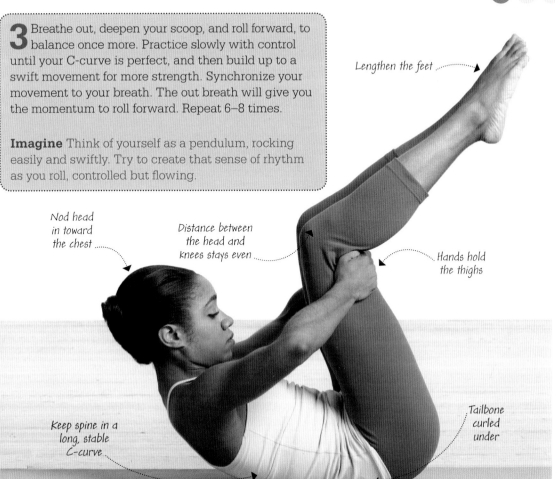

3 Breathe out, deepen your scoop, and roll forward, to balance once more. Practice slowly with control until your C-curve is perfect, and then build up to a swift movement for more strength. Synchronize your movement to your breath. The out breath will give you the momentum to roll forward. Repeat 6–8 times.

Imagine Think of yourself as a pendulum, rocking easily and swiftly. Try to create that sense of rhythm as you roll, controlled but flowing.

Lengthen the feet

Nod head in toward the chest

Distance between the head and knees stays even

Hands hold the thighs

Keep spine in a long, stable C-curve

Tailbone curled under

Take care...

Don't tilt your head back. If the eye-focus floats to the ceiling, the head will rock back. Keep your eyes focused into your center, chin nodding toward the chest.

Don't lose the C-curve and flatten the spine. Keep the abdominals constantly scooping in more deeply to strengthen the C-curve throughout the movement.

What not to do

Do not look up at the ceiling

Back should not be flat

Single Leg Stretch 1
Strengthen Stomach and Thighs
Practice Flowing Movement and Concentration
This is one of the most effective tummy-toning exercises you can do.
Focus on alignment and control, as you flow swiftly from a strong center.

1 Lie in the center of your mat. Float your knees into your chest and wrap your hands around your right knee. Breathe in and curl your head and shoulders off the mat, simultaneously reaching your left leg away.

Tip To help you keep the curl-up position, aim your gaze between your thighs, belly deeply scooped. Do not lose the curl-up.

Bring the knee in toward the forehead

Reach the leg straight and strong

Pull the leg in strongly, using your arms

2 As you breathe out, draw the leg in and switch the arm and leg positions. Breathe in to extend the left leg, and out to extend the right leg. Repeat up to 8 times on each leg.

Careful! Stay central and keep the torso controlled. Think about your box (see p.30).

Take care...

Don't drop your head back, so your eye-focus floats up. This places strain on the neck. Keep the eyes focused down toward the pelvis.

Make sure your head is centered on the spine as the limbs move. The head should remain still: think of your box square and even.

Try not to collapse the knee into the chest. Keep it precise.

What not to do

Don't allow your head to drop back

Double Leg Stretch 1

Strengthen Stomach and Buttocks • **Practice** Centering

Lengthening your limbs away from your center is a real test of your core strength and control. Keep in mind all the Pilates principles—this exercise will really challenge you.

1 Lie on your back, float your knees into your chest, and hug them in using your hands. On an out breath, curl your head toward your knees.

Tip Draw in your belly, scooping it away from your nose. Keep the shoulders relaxed.

Look down toward your navel

Scoop the belly

Neck is long and relaxed

Shins parallel with the floor, feet pointed

2 Breathe in and stretch your arms forward. Check that your scoop stays deep and the lower back sinks toward the mat.

Help! If your neck strains, place one hand behind your head.

3 Stretch your legs away. Squeeze the inner thighs and deepen your scoop. Breathe out, hug the knees in, then repeat without curling back down. Repeat 6–8 times.

Careful! Don't allow the back to arch. Take the legs only as low as you can control them.

Eyes focused forward

Sink the belly into the lower spine

Legs squeezed in Pilates stance

Spine Stretch Forward 1

Strengthen Back and Stomach • **Practice** Breathing

This will test your C-curve (see p.36) and strengthen the abdominals and the spine. It's also a wonderful way of stretching the back and hamstrings, and making you aware of your posture.

1 Sit tall, with your legs lengthened, slightly wider than hip-width apart. Press your hands into the mat, in between your legs. Feel your shoulder blades soften back. Lengthen the rib cage up, away from the hips.

Tip Check the entire body is active and you'll feel the exercise more effectively. Press out through the feet and feel the crown of the head lengthen upward. Imagine your spine is like a spring, reaching and stretching.

Lift your belly and lengthen your waist

Press out through the heels

2 As you breathe out, nod the chin to the chest, and curl your spine into a C-curve. Nod the crown of the head forward. Hold the arches of the feet. Breathe in and stretch the spine and legs. As you breathe out, slowly re-stack the spine, using your abdominals. Press the palms into the floor once more. Repeat up to 5 times. Stay lifted in the abdominals and waist. Sit taller as you re-stack to an upright position.

Imagine As you pull forward toward your feet, imagine there is a belt pulling your waist back.

Keep the neck long

Tilt the head forward

Belly lifts back to lengthen the spine

Keep pressing out through the feet

Spine Twist

Strengthen Waist and Spine • **Practice** Precision

This exercise requires precision and control. The muscles on both sides of the body are equally challenged to produce the twisting movement, therefore toning the waist.

1 Sit tall, legs connected, hands clasped behind your head. Press out through the heels and draw the belly up and in. Breathe in and lengthen the spine.

Imagine To keep your back straight, imagine sitting tall with your spine lined up against a pole.

Press the head into the hands to lengthen the spine

Squeeze the inner thighs

The elbows stay wide and open

Stay lifted with the torso; don't lean forward or back

Press out through the heels

2 Breathe out and twist the spine to the right, keeping the pelvis square. Lift up through the crown of the head. Reach your left elbow forward and the right elbow back, keeping the chest open.

Imagine As you twist, think of the rib cage spiraling around the spine, growing taller.

3 Breathe in to return to the center, then breathe out to twist to the other side. Repeat 6 times on each side.

Tip Keep the spine lifting tall as you twist and the muscles will have to work harder. Imagine sending the rib cage back behind you, keeping the elbows wide.

Relax the shoulders into the back

Lift the waist up with each twist

Keep the lower back long, don't curl the tailbone

Tick Tock

Strengthen Waist and Inner Thighs
Practice Control and Concentration

Control this movement and your abdominals will soon be well
toned. Move slowly at first and gradually increase the range,
until you can reach the legs lower with control.

1 Lie flat, fold your knees in, and lengthen the legs up to the ceiling, directly above the hips. Bring the legs into Pilates stance. Reach your arms out by your sides, pressing them into the floor to help ground the torso. Breathe in to prepare.

Help! If your legs cramp at 90°, bend the knees slightly.

Heels together, toes apart

Squeeze the inner thighs

Draw the belly in and up

2 Breathe out and lower the legs to the right. Ensure the legs are connected from the inner thighs to the heels. Feel the left side of your rib cage anchoring into the floor as the hips twist to the right. Breathe out to draw the legs back to center. Then breathe in to lower the legs to the left. Repeat up to 5 times on each side.

Tip Feel this twist coming from your navel, not from the hips. Go only as low as you can control with your abdominals.

Legs straight and level, squeezing together

Keep your eyes focused on the ceiling

Maintain a strong scoop

Keep the shoulders heavy

Swan Preparation

Strengthen Back • **Practice** Precision

This is a great way to counteract bad posture. It opens
out the chest and strengthens the muscles of the
mid-back and the upper arms.

1 Lie on your front, with legs together in parallel.
Place the hands directly beneath the shoulders and
draw your elbows in tightly to the waist, pointing
them back, as if you're a crocodile.

Careful! Try not to sink into and compress the lower
back. Always keep the stomach muscles lifted.

Arms squeezed in
toward the body

Legs in parallel,
tightly squeezed

2 Breathe in. As you breathe out, look up, glide the
shoulder blades back, and open your chest up.
Push the elbows down toward the floor. Hold for
5 breaths, keeping the belly lifted. Breathe out and
lower down to the mat slowly. Repeat 5 times.

Tip Activate the muscles in-between the shoulder
blades to lift the spine. Keep the neck long, throat open.

Relax the
shoulders down

Reach the
crown of the
head away

Reach the legs
with energy

Open the chest

Knee Stretches

Strengthen Stomach and Buttocks
Practice Control and Flowing Movement

Great for coordination and control, this exercise combines
flowing movement of the spine with reaching limbs away from
a strong center. It's a great way to focus the mind on your body.

1 Come onto all fours in the center of your mat. Think about your Pilates box, with long waist even on both sides. Draw the belly up away from the floor. Lengthen the spine into neutral. Spread the weight evenly through the hands. Breathe in to prepare.

Imagine Visualize yourself as a table, strong and sturdy, with your weight supported evenly through each limb.

Keep your spine flat, neither arched nor tucked under

Neck is long and in line with the spine

Feet lengthened and in parallel

Abdominals lift into the back

Use your buttock to draw the leg in

Keep the arms straight and strong

2 As you breathe out, curl the tailbone underneath you and roll the spine up into a C-curve. Simultaneously, bring the right knee in toward your forehead. Keep the belly lifted.

Careful! Try to stay centered on your mat. Try not to allow the body to lean and wobble as you move the leg. Stay strong and centered.

3 Breathe in and lengthen the right leg back behind you, keeping your hips square. Extend the spine and bring your gaze up. Increase the momentum and repeat 6–8 times on the right side, then shift to the left leg and perform the same number of repetitions.

Remember Alignment is key. Try not to allow the body to rock from side to side. Keep your box still as the leg reaches away.

Keep your head in line with the spine

Buttocks engaged

Lengthen the leg in line with the body

Feel the arms working

Keep your box square

Foot in line with the knee

Knee directly underneath the hip

Take care...

Don't take your leg up too high. Make sure you control the movement and keep the leg in line with the hip. Lifting too high will allow the back to arch.

Don't rock your body from side to side. Keep your core strong and stay central in your mat.

The opposite hip shouldn't drop as you bring the leg in. Use your powerhouse to stay level in the hips.

Increase the momentum gradually and always more precisely. Try not to swing your whole body with the leg. Keep the abdominals strong to control the movement.

Side Kicks: Front 1

Strengthen Waist and Buttocks • **Practice** Centering

This tones the waist and buttocks, challenging your balance
and control. When performing the Side Kick series (see pp.72–75),
repeat all exercises on one side before rolling over and
repeating the entire sequence on the other side.

1 Lie down on your side, legs straight and at about
45°, hips and shoulders stacked on top of each other.
Scoop the belly in, lengthening the waist. Rest your
head on your hand. Place your top hand on the mat in
front of your rib cage.

Tip Release the arm and rest it on the floor, and relax
your head onto your arm.

Reach the head
actively away

Head presses
into the hand,
neck long

Lift the underside
of your waist

Legs squeezing
in Pilates stance

2 Breathe out, lift the top leg, in line with the hip.
Keep the waist long and belly deeply scooped. Try
to make the top leg longer than the bottom leg, and
remember to move with length.

Reach your top
leg longer than
the bottom leg

Draw the belly
in tightly

Keep
shoulders
open

3 Breathe in and swing your leg forward, then pulse forward twice by pushing your leg forward and back a little bit more in small, heartbeat movements. Ensure the tailbone doesn't curl forward with the thighbone. Keep the leg lifted and parallel with the floor.

Imagine Visualize sliding your leg along a table, staying on exactly the same level throughout.

Take care...

Don't swing your spine with the leg. Make sure your bottom doesn't curl under as the leg comes forward. Keep your core strong so the spine is stable and resists movement.

Keep the head pressed into your hand

Slide the leg forward without dipping

Actively reach the lower leg away

4 Breathe out, sweep the top leg back, opening the front of the hip. Make sure the knee doesn't bend. Repeat 6–8 times on this side, then roll over and repeat on the other side.

Careful! Make sure the spine doesn't swing with the leg. Keep your powerhouse working.

Reach outward through the crown of the head

Shoulders soft into the back

Keep the legs turned out of the hip and buttocks working

Keep the knees straight

Side Kicks: Double Leg Lift

Strengthen Inner Thighs, Buttocks, and Waist
Practice Precision

Working your waist and thighs, this adds a little more
challenge to your Side Kick series. Think about balance
and control, and the precision and pacing of the movement.

1 Lie on your side with your legs still forward by
about 45°. Use the mat as a guide for your
alignment. Lengthen your feet toward the front of the
mat. Place the legs in Pilates stance. Breathe in.

Tip Focus on length, reaching the legs away from the
crown of the head. Keep the abdominals working hard.

Relax the
shoulder
into the back

Keep the neck
long and head
pressing into
the hands

Squeeze the heels
in Pilates stance

2 Breathe out, lift and lengthen both legs up, with
inner thighs squeezing and reaching away through
the toes. Breathe in. Breathe out and release the legs
down slowly. Repeat up to 8 times on each side.

Tip Lift the legs only as high as you can.

Keep the
shoulder
relaxed

Lengthen the
head away
from the spine

Keep the waist long

Maintain
your Pilates
stance

Side Kicks: Lower Lift

Strengthen Core • **Practice** Concentration

Concentrate on your alignment and coordination for this
exercise, working the targeted areas while keeping the rest
of your body long and free from tension.

1 Lie on your mat. Breathe in to prepare and
lengthen your spine. Keep the waist long on
both sides and engage the belly muscles strongly.
Breathe out to lift both legs together, squeezing the
buttocks and thighs.

Tip Keep the waist long to avoid slumping into the mat.

Look directly
forward

The forearm
takes the weight
of the head

Legs squeezing in
Pilates stance

2 Breathe in and lower the bottom leg toward the
floor, then breathe out to lift it again, squeezing
the inner thighs and heels. Lift and lower up to 10
times, lifting with the out breath and deepening
the abdominals. Release both legs down together.
Repeat up to 8 times.

Lengthen
and reach
out through
the crown of
the head

Relax the
shoulders

Keep the top leg
lifted and still

Mermaid

Strengthen Waist and Core
Practice Centering and Flowing Movement

This is a lovely stretch after the Side Kicks series—to stretch the waist—creating space in your spine, and working on flow.

1 Sit tall with your legs curled to one side and knees level. Try to feel evenly grounded through both the sit bones and lifted through your waist. Breathe in and float one arm up in line with the ear, and take the other around the shins. Think about lifting your rib cage up and away from the hips throughout. Stay square and try not to allow the box to collapse.

Careful! If you have knee problems, you need to avoid this exercise because it might put pressure on the knee joints.

Palm facing in, fingers long

Relax the shoulder away from the ear

Arm open, hand resting on the shin

Keep the pelvis square

Keep the shoulder away from the ear

Reach the hand long

Stretch the waist

Feet stacked on top of each other

2 Breathe out; reach the arm up and over the body, lengthening both sides of the waist. Breathe in to use your powerhouse.

Imagine As you reach your arm up, imagine you are painting a line on the ceiling above you with your fingertips.

Careful! Make sure you don't collapse the bottom side of the waist. The obliques should lift the rib cage throughout.

3 Float back to the center with your out breath. Lengthen the spine and relax the shoulders. Keep your gaze forward to ensure the head is in line with the spine; don't tilt the head down.

Tip Feel the spine lifting up before it bends. Create a space between each vertebra.

Reach the arm straight to the ceiling

Relax the shoulder

Keep hips square

Feet stay together

Reach the arm up and away

Keep the elbow in line with the ear

Keep looking forward

Keep the rib cage lifted toward the ceiling

Press the hand into the mat

Keep the hip on the mat

4 Breathe out to place the arm down onto the mat, bending the elbow. Float the other arm up and across. Repeat 3 times on each side. The legs remain still and anchored as the body floats gracefully as if under water.

Remember It should be a graceful, flowing movement. Stay lifted in the waist throughout.

Take care...

Don't collapse your chest. Keep the shoulders open, as if you are sliding between two panes of glass.

Don't keep your eyes focused downward. Make sure you look straight ahead throughout the movement and keep the neck in line with the spine.

What not to do

Don't collapse your chest

Don't bend the arm over the head

Shoulder Bridge

Strengthen Buttocks and Core • **Practice** Control

This exercise tones the buttocks and builds your strength and stamina. Imagine you are under water, and use the resistance to make your movements precise. Hold the pelvis lifted and stable, as you move the legs with control.

1 Lie on your back with your arms relaxed by your sides. Your legs are hip-width apart, feet flat on the floor. Your spine is in neutral, powerhouse engaged. Breathe in to prepare.

Point the knees toward the ceiling

Relax the shoulders

Keep the feet flat on the floor

2 Breathe out and hinge the hips up in one movement. Keep the rib cage connected to avoid arching the back. Shoulders are heavy and open, arms pressing into the floor. Hold this position for 5 breaths. Release the spine back down, then move on to step 3.

Connect the rib cage into the waist

Engage the buttocks to press the hips up

3 Hinge the hips up once again. Extend your right leg up to the ceiling, foot softly pointed. Make sure your hips stay level and lifted, your box strong. Feel heavy and grounded through the supporting foot.

Reach the leg straight up to the ceiling

Keep the bottom lifted

Press the supporting foot down

4 Breathe in and kick the leg down, flexing the foot. Repeat steps 3 and 4 five times. Breathe out for up-kick and in for down-kick, then float the foot down, keeping the hips lifted. Repeat with the other leg.

Maintain a strong center to avoid arching the back

Take care...

Don't drop the hips on one side. Think about your box and keep it square and lifted.

Don't lift the shoulders. Keep your shoulders released heavily into the floor.

Check your foot isn't too close to your bottom. Keep it in line with the knee, so the spine can lengthen.

What not to do

Leg is bent

Supporting foot close to the bottom

Spine has arched

15-Minute Sequence

1 Pilates Stance p.35

2 Wall: Roll Down pp.42–43

3 Standing Side Bends p.51

6 Leg Circles pp.60–61

7 Rolling Like a Ball 1 pp.62–63

10 Spine Stretch Forward 1 p.66

11 Spine Twist p.67

4 Hundred Preparation
pp.54–55

5 Roll Back
pp.56–57

8 Single Leg Stretch 1
p.64

9 Double Leg Stretch 1
p.65

12 Swan Preparation
p.69

13 Mermaid
pp.76–77

30-Minute Sequence

1 **Pilates Stance** p.35

2 **Wall: Roll Down** p.42

3 **Wall: Stand** p.44

7 **Pelvic Curls** p.39

8 **Hundred Preparation** pp.54–55

9 **Roll Back** pp.56–57

13 **Single Leg Stretch 1** p.64

14 **Double Leg Stretch 1** p.65

15 **Spine Stretch Forward 1** p.66

19 **Swan Preparation** p.69

20 **Mermaid** pp.76–77

4 Wall: Chair
p.45

5 Standing Side Bends
p.51

6 Neck Presses
p.38

10 Roll Up
pp.58–59

11 Leg Circles
pp.60–61

12 Rolling Like a Ball 1
pp.62–63

16 Spine Twist
p.67

17 Knee Stretches
pp.70–71

18 Side Kicks: Front 1
pp.72–73

45-Minute Sequence

1 **Pilates Stance**
p.35

2 **Wall: Roll Down**
p.42

3 **Wall: Stand**
p.44

7 **Neck Presses**
p.38

8 **Pelvic Curls**
p.39

9 **Seated C-curve**
p.36

13 **Leg Circles**
pp.60–61

14 **Rolling Like a Ball 1**
pp.62–63

15 **Single Leg Stretch 1**
p.64

19 **Knee Stretches**
pp.70–71

20 **Side Kicks: Front 1**
pp.72–73

21 **Side Kicks: Double Leg Lift**
p.74

25 **Swan Preparation**
p.69

26 **Mermaid**
pp.76–77

27 **Wall: Circles**
pp.46–47

4

Wall: Chair
p.45

5 Standing Side
Bends
p.51

6 Powerhouse
p.37

10 Hundred
Preparation
pp.54–55

11 Roll Back
pp.56–57

12 Roll Up
pp.58–59

16 Double Leg Stretch 1
p.65

17 Spine Stretch
Forward 1
p.66

18 Spine Twist
p.67

22 Side Kicks:
Lower Lift
p.75

23 Tick Tock
p.68

24 Shoulder Bridge
pp.78–79

28

**Biceps: Front
Curls**
p.48

29

**Biceps:
Side Curls**
p.49

30 Boxing
p.50

Assess your progress

How did you progress over the last six weeks? Go back and check your baselines (see pp.28–29). How do you feel compared to the first time you performed the exercises? Did you notice an improvement? If so, well done! Keep at it!

Common problems

Did you make less progress than you'd hoped? Don't be disheartened. Look again at the sections on The 6 Principles of Pilates (see pp.8–11) and Key Techniques (see pp.30–39). Practice, practice, practice any key techniques that still don't make sense to you.

Be honest: Did you stick to the program and focus on each detail fully as you worked? Pilates is all about detail, so your progress directly reflects the effort and concentration you put into each workout. Here are some common problems that beginners face.

"My muscles quiver when I curl up from the mat or hold my legs in the air."

This is not unusual. My Pilates teacher called it "the tremor of truth!" It means your muscles are working hard. As long as you don't feel any strain or sharp pain, breathe through the wobbling; your muscles will soon respond and strengthen. Deepen the abdominal connection as you curl up or move the limbs. Relax rather than tense up.

"I find it hard to arch my back up from the mat."

Being unable to lengthen the spine up from a face-down position, such as in Swan Preparation (see p.69), shows a lack of spinal flexibility. It is very common for bad posture to cause weak spinal muscles. To encourage more mobility, focus on practicing this lying position, even if it feels uncomfortable (although never work through pain). Try to achieve even a small bending movement of the upper spine and aim to improve each time. Your mobility should increase, to benefit your posture and spinal health.

"My neck aches during the curl-up exercises."

Check your eye focus during these exercises. When abdominals tire, often you slightly lose your curl up and the head begins to drop back, so the eyes focus on the ceiling. This strains the neck muscles, causing an ache. Relax the head down whenever you feel this ache. To avoid it, deepen your powerhouse connection (see p.37). Make sure that your belly stays strong to the end of an exercise and keep your eyes focused toward your center to keep the neck free and long.

"I can't straighten my legs."

Tight muscles respond very well to regular stretching. Continue with the program: Soften your knees if it is uncomfortable, but try to push yourself slightly to straighten a little farther each time. Your hamstrings will soon begin to lengthen.

"Pilates is too easy! This is boring."

Quite simply, if you find Pilates easy you are not working hard enough. Even the key techniques can offer as much challenge as you wish to take from them, so make the most of each exercise. Strive to perform each one precisely. Don't rush, really feel it: Work slowly, with control, thinking about precision, lengthening, breathing, alignment, scoop, and coordination....

Assess your achievement

Didn't achieve your goals? Don't allow it to dampen your enthusiasm as you move to the next section (see pp.88–139). Celebrate every achievement as you practice, for example being able to coordinate your movement to your breath, or to straighten your leg slightly farther than before. Small results accumulate: Soon you'll be setting yourself new goals.

Challenging exercises

Here is a plan to help you during your workouts over the next six weeks. At the end of the six weeks, look back over these goals and assess how you have progressed.

Goal: Control
Roll Back (see pp.56–57)

Work on moving smoothly, with a strong core

Goal: Centering
Centering (see p.40)

Work on flowing movement from a strong core, keeping the spine still

Goal: Flexibility
Wall: Roll Down
(see pp.42–43)

Work on rolling the spine like a wheel, peeling each bone away individually

Goal: Strength
Wall: Chair (see p.45), Hundred Preparation (see pp.54–55), Roll Up (see pp.58–59)

Work on staying stable through each exercise, flowing each one to the next without a break

Goal: Flowing Movement
Single Leg Stretch 1 (see p.64)

Work on moving the limbs smoothly without stopping and starting

2

Build On It

Now that you've mastered the basics, you're ready to move on to more complex versions of some of the exercises, as well as some new ones. Continue to perfect the movements you already know and practice anything that you find challenging until you feel completely confident with each movement. Precision and concentration are key. After working through this chapter, you should find that you are performing the movement sequences with much more fluidity and control.

Plan Your Program

Well done for getting this far! By now you should feel stronger, more supple, and better coordinated. You may also feel that Pilates is becoming a part of your life and that you no longer have to think twice about scheduling workout time.

Planning the next step

Now we want to take the next steps into developing greater understanding of Pilates and really working our bodies harder to reach new goals with our newly acquired skills. Let's continue to use broadly the same goals as for the first stage, so that we can gain a real picture of how far we have come when we reach the end of this program. Once you have followed these sequences a few times, you could mix and match other exercises from the rest of the section—but make sure that any substitutions train the same area of the body, to ensure that your workout remains balanced.

Build On It Exercise Program

Use this specially designed Pilates exercise program (below and opposite) to set yourself goals and assess your progress over the next six weeks. You can find summaries of the sequences on pp.132–137. Each week, when you work out, follow the sequence provided in this program at least for the first few times, before you experiment with using other exercises on the same level. Remember to act as your own coach and don't allow yourself to be lazy or cheat—you will improve more quickly if you perform every movement to the best of your ability.

Week 1: Focus on Alignment

Baseline: The original photographs you took at the start of the Start Simple Exercise Program (see pp.28–29).
- **Day 1:** 15-minute sequence, check control, breathing
- **Day 2:** 30-minute sequence, check lengthening, stability
- **Day 3:** 45-minute sequence, check precision, control
- **Day 4:** 15-minute sequence, check stability, coordination

Goal: Take new photos after six weeks to see how much closer you are to ideal alignment.

Week 2: Focus on Control

Baseline: Perform the Teaser with Twist (see pp.126–127). Do you feel stiff and wobbly? Can you hold the position without shaking or tensing? Do you collapse in the spine or can you maintain length and height as you twist?
- **Day 1:** 15-minute sequence, check centering, alignment
- **Day 2:** 45-minute sequence, check concentration, precision
- **Day 3:** 15-minute sequence, check precision, breathing
- **Day 4:** 45-minute sequence, check flowing movement, stability

Goal: Do the exercise with control, precision, and fluidity, feeling strong and supported as you twist.

Week 3: Focus on Centering
Baseline: Perform Double Leg Stretch 2 (see pp.102–103). Does your spine arch as you lengthen the limbs away? Are the shoulders away from the ears? Is the spine supported and strong, or does the lower back feel weak?
- **Day 1:** 15-minute sequence, check Pilates box, alignment, flowing movement
- **Day 2:** 30-minute sequence, check stability, precision, lengthening
- **Day 3:** 45-minute sequence, check precision, control, breathing
- **Day 4:** 30-minute sequence, check control, alignment.

Goal: Hold a strong center as you lengthen the limbs, with no movement in the spine.

Week 4: Focus on Flexibility
Baseline: Perform Single Straight Leg Stretch (see p.101). Are you able to straighten your legs up to the ceiling?
- **Day 1:** 15-minute sequence, check precision, control, alignment
- **Day 2:** 45-minute sequence, check breathing, scoop, stability
- **Day 3:** 45-minute sequence, check scoop, powerhouse, coordination
- **Day 4:** 30-minute sequence, check control, concentration.

Goal: Lengthen and straighten the legs without wobbling.

Week 5: Focus on Strength
Baseline: Try performing Ten by Ten (see pp.92–93), Half Roll Up (see pp.94–95), Teaser Preparation (see pp.124–125) without a break. On a scale of 1–10, how hard was each exercise and the sequence?
- **Day 1:** 15-minute sequence, check centering, control, coordination
- **Day 2:** 45-minute sequence, check scoop, alignment, concentration
- **Day 3:** 30-minute sequence, check alignment, coordination, flowing movement
- **Day 4:** 45-minute sequence, check control, precision, powerhouse

Goal: When you do the sequence again, it should feel easier.

Week 6: Focus on Flowing Movement
Baseline: Try Swimming (see pp.128–129). Does the movement feel fluid and controlled or jerky? Can you link leg and arm movements simultaneously without stopping the flow?
- **Day 1:** 30-minute sequence, check centering, breathing, coordination
- **Day 2:** 45-minute sequence, check stability, control, Pilates box
- **Day 3:** 30-minute sequence, check alignment, precision, coordination
- **Day 4:** 45-minute sequence, check precision, centering, breathing

Goal: Make the movement smoother and swifter without wobbling or stopping.

Check your new baseline for each area of the body before you begin this exercise program and make a note of how it feels to do each movement. Then, at the end of the six weeks, assess yourself, according to the goals given here, to see how far you have gone toward achieving your targets. Enjoy the next six weeks!

Ten by Ten

Strengthen Stomach • **Practice** Breathing

This exercise builds your strength for the full Hundred (see p.144).
It warms up the body, works the powerhouse, and uses the
Pilates breath wide into the back of the body. It should appear
effortless, not labored, as you work the muscles hard.

1 Sit tall, with your knees connected, feet flat on the floor. Reach your arms out in front, shoulders soft into your back. Breathe out to scoop the belly, curl the tailbone under, and begin to release the spine, bone by bone, into the mat. Maintain a strong engagement of your abdominals.

Tip Relax the shoulders and keep them connected into your body as your arms reach away.

Reach the arms parallel with the legs

Keep the belly scooped

Keep the shoulders soft and relaxed

Squeeze the inner thighs

Keep the upper body lifted

2 Release down until you reach the tips of your shoulder blades. Your spine is curled, arms reaching away parallel with your thighs. Lengthen the right leg away from the knee, keeping the inner thighs parallel and glued together. Press the supporting foot into the ground. Squeeze deeply into the belly to keep stable.

Careful! As you reach the leg away, deepen the scoop of your belly and keep the spine lifted. Try not to collapse your form.

3 Extend the left leg to meet the right. Breathe in, and pump the arms up and down—breathe in for 5 pumps and breathe out for 5. Then remain still and strong to breathe in for a count of 5 and out for 5. Alternate pumping and remaining still, and continue to breathe and pump in sets of 5 until you've reached 100.

Tip Feel light in the spine and move freely in the shoulder joints. Deepen the abdominals and imagine the rest of your body is serene as you dynamically pump the arms.

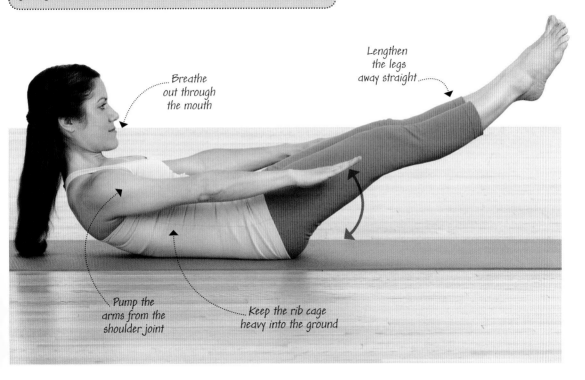

Breathe out through the mouth

Lengthen the legs away straight

Pump the arms from the shoulder joint

Keep the rib cage heavy into the ground

Take care...

Your neck shouldn't feel too strained. Your abdominals will get fatigued and need to be activated constantly. Keep your curl deep and powerhouse connected.

Don't move your torso. Move your shoulder joints without rocking the spine forward and back. Turn up your powerhouse engagement to keep the spine still.

Arms and hands shouldn't be floppy. Keep arms strong and straight from shoulder to fingertips. The pump is from the shoulder, not from the elbow, wrist, or fingers. Don't allow the arms to break at the wrist or the fingers to float. Reach out with energy through the fingertips as if you are bobbing a ball underneath your hands.

Half Roll Up

Strengthen Stomach
Practice Flowing Movement and Control

Make sure you move correctly in this exercise, using your
deep abdominals rather than lurching the spine up
or allowing other muscles to overwork.

1 Sit tall, then use your belly to curl your upper body over your legs, reaching the arms in line with the legs. Your nose reaches down toward your knees. Flex the feet away. Keep the belly lifted in and up. Imagine your spine lengthening like a spring.

Why? Flexing the feet ensures the legs are long and active, stretching the back of the thigh and providing a balance to the upper body as it moves.

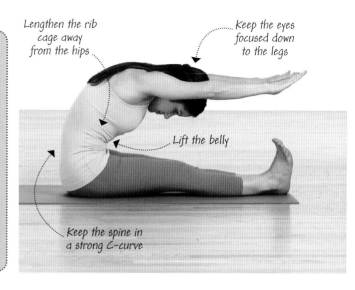

Lengthen the rib cage away from the hips

Keep the eyes focused down to the legs

Lift the belly

Keep the spine in a strong C-curve

Reach the arms away with energy

Keep the belly scooped

Soften the knees, but keep the legs lengthening away

2 Breathe in deeply as you start to roll your spine beneath you, controlling with your abdominals to release bone by bone toward the mat. Roll as far as you are able to control the movement, and hold it there for 3 breaths. Deeply engage the abdominals, and relax the shoulders and neck.

Remember Control is key. Make sure you go only as far as you are able to control the movement. Build up your strength slowly. Each time, go a little farther as your strength develops.

3 As you breathe out, deepen your scoop and squeeze the inner thighs and buttocks as you begin to roll back up and over the legs once more. Repeat 5 times. Each time, try to challenge yourself a little bit more to roll deeper, with control. Moving very slowly means you need to work the muscles harder because you can't rely on momentum.

Imagine Length is very important here. Imagine each bone of your spine reaching away from the one before it, lifting like bubbles as you move forward.

Stay lifted with the rib cage

Reach long through the fingertips

Feel the buttocks working

Take care...

Don't hold your breath. Make sure you keep breathing. When you are holding the position, deepen your abdominals further with each out breath, and check that the rest of your body is free from tension: jaw, neck, and shoulders.

Don't hunch your shoulders. Keep them soft and connected into the body as you curl.

Don't lift the feet. Stay heavy and grounded through the feet.

Mini Bridge

Strengthen Buttocks and Arms • **Practice** Concentration

This variation on the Shoulder Bridge (see pp.78–79) is great for building strength in your back and concentrating on your body. You use your body weight as resistance to build strength.

1 Align yourself centrally on your mat, legs lengthened on the floor with your feet flexed, arms relaxed by your sides, palms down. Breathe in to prepare and lengthen the spine.

Press down through the heels

Squeeze the legs together

Scoop the belly

Keep the shoulders open, arms released

Press the hands into the floor

2 Breathe out, engage the powerhouse, and press the hips up, lifting the buttocks off the mat. Feel the shoulders, arms, and heels pressing actively into the floor. Squeeze the legs strongly from the big-toe joints to the inner thighs. Hold for 5 breaths, not allowing the hips to drop. Slowly lower back down. Repeat 3 times.

Keep the ribs soft into the body

Reach the legs away

Flex the feet

Lift the bottom

Letter T

Strengthen Upper back • **Practice** Flowing Movement

Great for your posture, this exercise strengthens the muscles between the shoulder blades and tones the arms and shoulders, too. To add a challenge, hold hand weights in each hand.

1 Lie on your front, legs together and in parallel. Engage your powerhouse to peel the front of the body off the mat, reaching the arms out to the sides, in line with your shoulders. Keep your eyes focused down toward the mat, and the neck long. Breathe in to prepare and lengthen the spine.

Lengthen the neck at the end of the spine

Reach the legs away

Palms face down

2 Breathe out to float the arms behind you and toward each other, reaching away with fingertips, lifting your chin and chest. Feel the shoulder blades gliding into the back. Breathe in to float back slowly to the start position. Repeat 5 times.

Reach with the arms, keeping the palms down

Keep the toes lengthening away

Keep the eyes focused forward

Shoulders stay away from the ears, neck long

Rolling Like a Ball 2

Strengthen Stomach • **Practice** Breathing

Use your powerhouse to maintain a C-curve and move
with flow and control. This is a playful exercise, suggesting
the joy and freedom of the movement of a child.

1 While sitting, create a C-curve with your spine. Fold the knees in toward your forehead, keeping them hip-width apart. Hold the ankles in your hands, feet together. Tip back off your sit bones, float the feet off the ground, and look down toward your navel. Deepen the scoop of your belly, hold your legs in tight to create a ball shape. Maintain this position throughout.

Why? The deep abdominal scoop is needed to create a C-shape and support the spine to prevent unwanted movement.

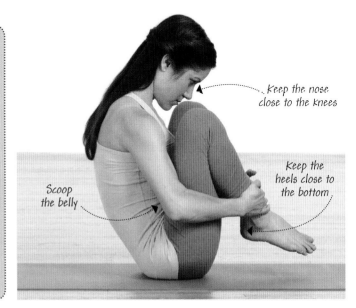

Keep the nose close to the knees

Keep the heels close to the bottom

Scoop the belly

Pull the feet in tight, heels close to the bottom

Direct the nose in to the belly

Roll through the lower back

2 Breathe in to roll back, maintaining the C-curve using your abdominals. You should feel each vertebra rolling evenly. Make sure your position does not change as you are rolling back. Keep the eye-focus in toward your center. Stay in a strong C-curve.

Imagine To help maintain the position, imagine an unbreakable magnetic connection between your heels and your bottom, and your nose and your belly.

3 Roll all the way back to the shoulder blades, no farther, sending your tailbone to the ceiling. Breathe out and roll back to the start position. Repeat up to 10 times, balancing momentarily between each roll. Keep your C-curve position throughout.

Help! If this feels very difficult, go back to your seated C-curve (see p.63) and really try to maintain this position as you roll. It takes time, but practice makes perfect!

Hands keep the shins in tightly

Knees reach in toward the forehead

Raise your tailbone toward the ceiling

Maintain your C-curve

Take care...

Don't roll your head back, keep it focused between the knees. If you look up, your back will straighten and you will end up stranded on the mat like a beetle on its back, unable to roll back up.

Try not to lose the C-curve. Don't allow the back to straighten when you reach the top of the roll. Keep the belly working when you balance at the end.

Your heels should not kick up to the ceiling. Keep the shins tightly drawn in toward you to avoid kicking the legs up. Maintain your ball shape throughout.

Keep the flow. This movement should be brisk and continuous. Ensure you breathe in to roll back, out to roll forward, and keep the momentum going.

Single Leg Stretch 2

Strengthen Stomach • **Practice** Precision

This version of Single Leg Stretch 1 (see p.64) requires more focus as you pick up speed and coordinate your hand and leg movements. Work hard on maintaining a strong, stable torso.

1 Curl up, hugging your right knee into your chest. Put your right hand on your right ankle, and left hand across the knee. Reach your left leg away, in line with the body, and as low as you can take it without losing control of your spine. Breathe in to prepare.

Place your right hand on the ankle

Place your left hand on the knee

Press the leg away against resistance

2 Breathe out to switch legs and swap hand positions. Continue to alternate, breathing in to lengthen one leg and breathing out to return and lengthen the other. With each movement, maintain your deep belly scoop throughout.

Keep the elbows wide

Keep looking into your center

Relax the shoulders

Single Straight Leg Stretch

Strengthen Stomach • **Practice** Flowing Movement

Also known as "scissors," this exercise requires controlled, brisk movements that work your core and dynamically stretch the hamstrings.

1 Lie on your back, with the box square on the mat. Hug your knees to your chest and curl your forehead to your knees. Reach your right leg up to the ceiling and hold the ankle with both hands. Reach your left leg out in front of you. Turn the legs out in Pilates stance. Breathe out to pulse twice quickly, with the right leg stretching the hamstring as you draw the leg in toward your head.

Imagine Think of it as a heartbeat, rhythmically pulling the leg in twice, then pressing away.

Reach the opposite leg away with energy

Keep the leg long and straight as you pull it toward you

Keep your center working throughout

Keep the elbows soft

Make sure the shoulders are relaxed into the body

2 Breathe in to swap the leg positions, then pulse twice with the left leg while breathing out. Switch legs rapidly, keeping the torso absolutely still as you scissor the legs in and out. Repeat 8 times on each leg.

Careful! Keep the powerhouse working to ensure the body does not rock or bounce with the leg movement.

Double Leg Stretch 2

Strengthen Stomach • **Practice** Centering

This version of Double Leg Stretch 1 requires more control and strength (see p.65). As you lengthen all four limbs away from the center, you must maintain a stable spine. Be careful not to arch the back.

1 Lie flat, hugging the knees in toward your chest, taking the hands around the shins. Breathe out, use your abs and curl up, looking in toward your navel. Deepen your abdominal connection and feel the lower back releasing toward the mat.

Help! If your neck feels strained, do this exercise with your hands behind the head until you have the abdominal strength.

Keep the shins parallel to the floor

Release the spine into the mat, using your belly scoop

...Take the arms as far as you can

Squeeze the legs as you extend them

Keep the rib cage down

Keep the abdominals solid

2 Breathe in and reach the arms behind you, in line with your ears, while you simultaneously press the legs away, squeezing the legs together in Pilates stance. Sink your abdominals into the spine as you reach the limbs away.

Imagine To maintain this position, imagine your spine is anchored, so there is no movement as you reach the limbs away.

3 Breathe out, open the arms out to the sides and down toward the hips, extending the fingertips forward. Bend the knees in to return to the start position. Stay curled up, and repeat up to 6 times.

Careful! Precision is the key. Make sure you control the movement of the limbs and only take them within a safe range of movement for your spine. Build up your strength gradually.

Keep your legs in Pilates stance

Sink your belly deeper as you reach the limbs away

Keep the neck long

Reach the arm out freely from the shoulder joint

Use your belly to release the back into the floor

Take care...

Don't let the head fall back as you reach the arms and legs away. Make sure you maintain your curl, and keep the eyes focused downward as the arms stretch back.

Don't let the rib cage move. Keep it locked in position as the arms move fluidly.

Avoid arching the lower back as the legs release forward. Keep the belly strong to make sure the lower spine is heavy toward the mat. If necessary, keep the legs higher.

Don't let the arms carry the rib cage up. Stay strong in your center as you reach the arms freely behind you.

Spine Stretch Forward 2

Strengthen Stomach • **Practice** Breathing

A progression from stage 1 (see p.66), this version challenges your abdominals further by adding the weight of your arms to the movement. Focus on perfecting your C-curve.

Reach the crown of your head toward the ceiling

Keep the palms facing together

Close the ribs

Press the legs away, knees facing up from the floor

1 Sit tall on your mat, with your legs in parallel, slightly wider than hip-width apart and heels pressing away. Float the arms above you, in line with the ears. Lift the belly in and up. Breathe in to prepare.

Imagine Your pelvis is anchored into the ground, and your spine is light, like a balloon lifting up away from the anchored sit bones.

Lift the rib cage up away from the thighs

Draw the shoulders back into the body

Reach the arms in line with the legs

Engage the buttocks as you press the feet forward

2 Breathe out, lift the spine up as you roll forward, releasing the crown of the head toward your feet. Keep the arms in line with the ears and reach them over the feet. Deepen the abdominals. Keep the legs pressing away, activating the buttocks.

Imagine Picture someone pulling your waist back as you reach your fingertips forward.

Careful! Don't let the front of your body collapse as you curl forward. Lift even higher to resist the curl.

3 Breathe in and send the tailbone down to roll the spine back up sequentially. Float the arms up in line with the ears, shoulders relaxing into the back as you reach to the ceiling. Stay lifted through the abdominals and waist as you finish. Repeat 5 times.

Help! If you feel your shoulders hunching forward, connect your shoulder blades into the back and lengthen the neck, releasing the crown of the head forward.

Connect the shoulders down into the back

Reach the arms away

Lift the rib cage up, away from the hips

Take care...

Don't hinge at the hips. Make sure your abdominals create the movement by moving with an active C-curve of the spine.

Your legs should not be floppy. Check the legs are in parallel, heels pressing out and back of the legs active, as you curl forward and as you rebuild the spine.

Don't hunch your shoulders. Keep your neck long and feel your shoulder blades gliding into the back as you reach forward.

Don't collapse the front of the body. Resist gravity with your abdominals: lift up as you bend forward, as if someone has their hands around your waist from behind and is pulling your rib cage up.

Neck Roll

Strengthen Upper Back • **Practice** Control

An extension of the Swan Preparation (see p.69), this is a good stretch
for the abdominals, using a lot of abdominal control to support the
lower spine. When ready, you can move on to the Swan (see p.164).

Keep your head in line with the spine

Keep your lower back long, supported by your belly

1 Lie face down on the mat, legs connected. Keep the hands directly under the shoulders and elbows up toward the ceiling, hugging into your waist. Breathe in, lift your pelvic floor, and draw your belly in.

Draw the shoulders into the back

Reach the feet away actively

Keep the neck long

2 Breathe out, and roll the head and neck forward and up. Feel an even pressure into the hands as the elbows come toward the floor. Keep the shoulders soft into the back.

Keep the belly lifted away from the mat

Roll the neck to one side

3 Keep the belly scooped as you turn your gaze over one shoulder, to feel a gentle stretch in the neck. Keep your box square on the mat and avoid twisting the shoulders or ribs.

Keep the upper arms into the body

Reach the legs away

4 Circle the head down slowly to bring the chin toward the chest. Keep the torso lifted. Roll the neck across to the other side and look over that shoulder. Stay lengthened in the neck.

Careful! Maintain your powerhouse throughout to protect the lower back and to stop the belly dropping to the mat.

Feel the shoulder blades across the back

Keep the buttocks and thighs engaged

Softly point the feet

Spread the hands evenly

5 Bring your gaze back to the center, and then repeat to the other side. Make sure you stay lifted and strong throughout. Repeat twice in each direction.

Help! If you feel your shoulders or lower back straining, bring your arms slightly in front of you to relieve the pressure. If you feel the lower back sinking and straining, lift the belly in more.

Keep the neck long and reaching away from the torso

Keep the throat open

Keep the lower back long and supported by the belly

Keep the rib cage lifted

Magic Circle: Chest and Overhead

Strengthen Arms and Chest • **Practice** Control

This fabulous piece of equipment adds another dimension
to your practice. Here, you will tone the arms and shoulders.

Circle is directly in line with the chest

Relax shoulders into the back

Keep the neck long

Feel the shoulder blades connected into the back

Keep the palms long and active

Squeeze the buttocks and inner thighs

Draw the belly in and up

Draw the belly in and up, rib cage soft

Turn the legs out in Pilates stance

Keep the feet in Pilates stance

Chest Stand in Pilates stance. Hold the Circle in line with your chest. Press into the pads, fingers long. Breathe in. Stand tall, breathe out to compress the Circle, activating the shoulders. Hold for 3 counts, then release slowly with control. Repeat 5 times.

Overhead Stay lengthened and relaxed in the spine as you work the arms. Float the Circle above the head, keeping the arms slightly in front of you. Breathe out to press the pads of the Circle. Hold for 3 counts, then slowly release. Repeat 5 times.

Magic Circle: Pumping

Strengthen Arms and Shoulders • **Practice** Centering

Here you will add movement, so you need to flow and avoid
wobbling. Use your powerhouse to make sure the torso
is strong and stable as you move the arms.

Keep the wrists
long, in line
with the arms

Draw the belly
in strongly

Keep the legs
in Pilates stance

Lift the crown
of the head

Keep your
powerhouse
working

Pump from the
shoulder joint

Keep the
rib cage soft

Press with
long palms

Keep the feet in
Pilates stance

1 Stand in Pilates stance. Hold the
Circle out in front, at hip height. Keep
your arms extended and elbows soft.
Breathing naturally, pump the Circle 8 times
as you raise it above your head. Keep the
shoulders soft and down.

2 Pump 8 times to return to the start
position. Repeat 3 times. The arms
should float without affecting the position
of the shoulders or spine. Keep the spine
long and stable, eyes focused forward, and
legs squeezed together.

Magic Circle: Pliés

Strengthen Inner Thighs and Buttocks • **Practice** Control

A wonderful toner for the bottom and thighs, this balletic movement is great for your balance, too. Avoid this exercise if you have weak knees.

Keep the collarbones wide and the chest open

Relax the shoulders into the back

Squeeze with the inner thighs

Spread the feet in Pilates stance

Keep the elbows wide

Draw deeply into your center

Keep squeezing the buttocks

Bring the legs into a straightened position

1 Stand tall, with your hands on your hips. Keep the legs in Pilates stance and bent, knees directly over the toes. Place the Circle between the fleshy part of your thighs, just above the knees. Your spine should be long and neutral.

2 From your powerhouse, squeeze the Circle to straighten the legs. Hold the Circle steady and lengthen the crown of the head to the ceiling. Bend your knees back to the starting position and repeat the exercise 3–5 times.

Magic Circle: Inner Thighs and Arms

Strengthen Inner Thighs and Arms • **Practice** Concentration

These seated exercises require focus on your alignment
and posture. Engage your powerhouse throughout,
keeping the waist narrow and lifted.

Relax the shoulders away from the ears

Keep the waist long on both sides

Squeeze with the inner thighs

Place the feet in Pilates stance

Keep the neck long and relaxed

Press from the shoulder joints

Press down into the ball of the foot

Inner thighs Place the Circle between your thighs, feet flat on the floor. Fold your arms in front, shoulders relaxed. Lengthen the spine. Breathe out, squeeze from the powerhouse, holding for 3 counts as you breathe in. Relax, breathing out. Repeat 3–5 times.

Arms Hold the Circle out in front. Keep the legs parallel, hip-width apart. Lift your heels, pressing down into the balls of the feet and the toes. Squeeze the Circle between your palms, activating the chest and arms. Keep the spine long and neutral. Repeat 3–5 times.

Neck Pull

Strengthen Stomach • **Practice** Control

This is a tough yet rewarding exercise. You will need strong abdominals, because holding the arms behind the head places more load on those muscles. Try it with your arms crossed in front instead and feel the difference.

1 Sit tall, with legs out in front, hip-width apart and in parallel. Press out through the heels. Put your hands behind your head, placing one hand on top of the other. Lift into your center and lengthen the waist. Breathe in to hinge back from the hips.

Careful! If you feel this in the lower back as you hinge back, lift up your abdominals and engage the buttocks.

Open up and lift the chest

Draw deeply into your center, and be careful not to arch the back

Reach the toes to the ceiling

Feel the buttocks working

Lift the crown of the head to the ceiling

Keep the belly scooped

Press the heels forward

Reach the legs actively

2 Hinge to the lowest point you can without arching the back. Then breathe out to begin to curl the tailbone underneath you, nod the chin to the chest, and curl your spine into a C-curve, with waist lifted and long. Try to perform this movement perfectly.

Imagine Think of your spine as a spring, stretching and lengthening.

3 Continue to move while breathing out, the belly constantly lifted as you roll your spine forward, and send the nose over the knees. If you want to work harder, roll forward to a full spine stretch (see pp.104–105) with hands behind the head. Re-stack the spine tall and strong. Repeat 5 times.

Imagine Think of the rib cage being lifted to the ceiling; resist the pull with your muscles.

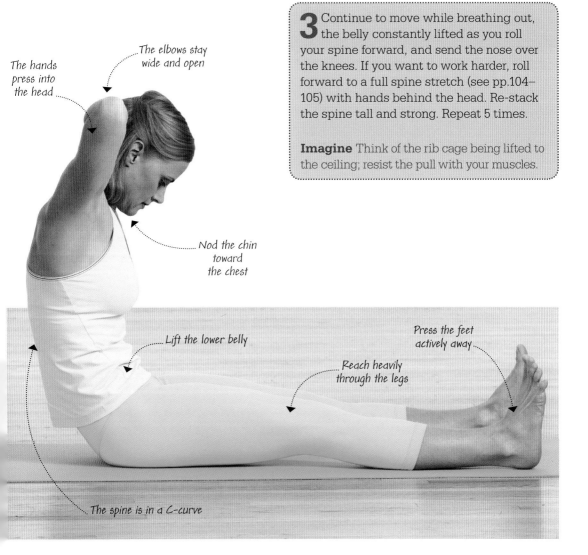

The hands press into the head

The elbows stay wide and open

Nod the chin toward the chest

Lift the lower belly

Press the feet actively away

Reach heavily through the legs

The spine is in a C-curve

Take care...

Try not to curl or arch your spine. Challenge your strength to hinge back as far as you can without curling the spine or arching. Keep the legs heavy and reaching away.

Don't lift and bend the legs as you hinge back. Make sure you actively reach away through the feet and imagine someone is sitting on your legs to weigh them down.

Don't let the abdominals collapse as you reach forward. Keep lifting continually throughout the exercise; never loosen the corset of muscles around the waist.

Don't hug your head with your elbows. Keep the elbows open and wide.

Side Kicks: Front 2

Strengthen Buttocks and Thighs • **Practice** Centering

Perform this series of Side Kick exercises on one side before moving to the other. This is more demanding than Side Kicks: Front 1 (see pp.72–73); you can't use your front arm for balance.

1 Lie on your left side, lined up with the back of the mat, shoulders and hips stacked. Place both hands behind your head. Press the head into the hands, with your neck lengthening and active. Hinge your hips forward so the legs aim toward the front corner of the mat. The legs are in parallel. Breathe in; lift the top leg.

Reach the crown of the head away

Make sure the waist is active and lifted

Flex the heels

Keep the top leg straight and level

Keep the bottom leg heavy and active

Take care...

Don't move the spine with the leg. Keep your powerhouse working hard. The leg should move independently from the spine, without taking the bottom with it.

Don't let your top shoulder drop forward. Use all your strength to resist the pull forward. Stay strong in your center and open in the chest.

Don't let the leg bend, drop, or lift at the knee. Lengthen it from the thighbone and keep it absolutely level.

2 Breathe out to swing the leg forward, pulsing it twice at the end of the swing. Keep the spine totally stable; resist the movement of bringing the tailbone under with the leg. Scoop the belly deeply throughout.

Help! Keep the swing small if your spine can't resist moving. Build it up until you can freely swing the leg without affecting the spine.

Keep the elbows open

Press the hands into the back of the head

Swing the leg on an even level

The bottom leg is reaching and heavy

3 Breathe in to sweep the leg back, taking it as far as you can to open the hip. Make sure the upper body does not collapse. Repeat up to 10 times. You can alternate flexing and pointing the foot.

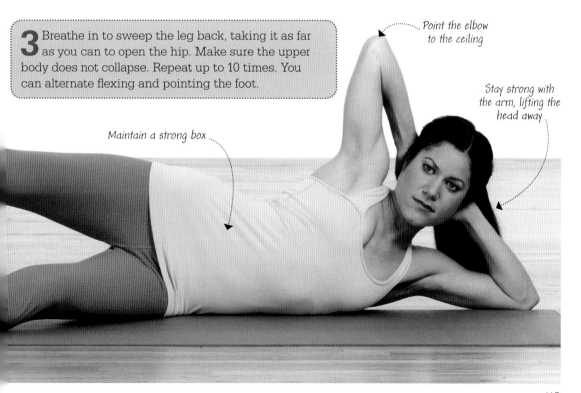

Point the elbow to the ceiling

Stay strong with the arm, lifting the head away

Maintain a strong box

Side Kicks: Scissors

Strengthen Back and Thighs
Practice Flowing Movement

This allows freedom of movement in the legs, working the
thigh and buttock muscles, and warming up the whole body.

1 Lie on your side, hand behind your head. Lift the
ribs. Rest the palm of your top hand on the mat in
front of your body for support. Squeeze your legs in
Pilates stance. Breathe in, and use your center to lift
and lengthen the legs to hip height.

Relax the
shoulder into
the back

Lengthen the crown
of the head away
from the spine

Connect the legs in
Pilates stance

Keep the legs in
Pilates stance
and straight

2 Breathe out to scissor the legs, taking the bottom leg forward first. Reach the legs equally behind and in front of you. Scissor the legs forward and back 6 times, maintaining a stable spine. Think about freeing the thigh joint, allowing mobility and fluidity with a strong, stable spine.

Careful! Don't forget to breathe throughout.

Take care...

Don't dip your waist into the mat. Resist the urge to slump the spine, stay strong and lifted in your abdominals.

Don't swing your back with the legs. Focus on your strong center and control the movement.

Don't let your head dip forward. Keep the front of your body open.

Point the feet softly in Pilates stance

Lengthen the waist

Press the head into the hand

Keep the legs long and straight

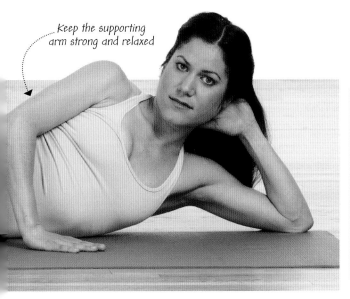

Keep the supporting arm strong and relaxed

3 Moving dynamically and breathing naturally, swing the legs for 6 more kicks, as swiftly as you can while controlling the movement. Keep checking your center is active.

Imagine The spine shouldn't move. Think of a thread linking the tailbone to the crown of the head and keeping your torso absolutely still.

Side Kicks: Circles

Strengthen Buttocks and Thighs • **Practice** Precision

The precision of this exercise will tone your buttocks
and thighs like nothing else. Make sure you keep
your alignment and powerhouse active.

1 Lie on your side, using your mat to guide your alignment, shoulders and hips stacked. Take your head in your hand; place the top hand in front. Bring the feet to the front of your mat, legs in Pilates stance. Lengthen the top leg to hip height, toes softly pointed.

Press the head into the hand

Keep the shoulder relaxed and open

Flex the bottom foot

Take care...

Don't let your upper body slump. Keep your powerhouse working and reach the neck active and long.

Don't just wiggle your toes. Make sure the circling movement is from the thighbone, as if you're turning a cocktail stick in a glass.

Don't allow the circles to be uneven, wobbly shapes. Keep the circles precise: really visualize them. This means your muscles will have to work harder.

Maintain the turnout of the leg

2 Breathe naturally as you circle the upper leg, keeping it in front of the bottom leg. The circles should be small, as if you're tracing the inside of a jam jar. Circle the leg 10 times.

Turn the leg out from the hip

Keep the belly strong

Turn the toes up to the ceiling

3 Lengthen the top leg back in line with the body, and circle 10 times again, behind the bottom leg. Keep the belly working to make sure the torso doesn't wobble as you circle from the thigh.

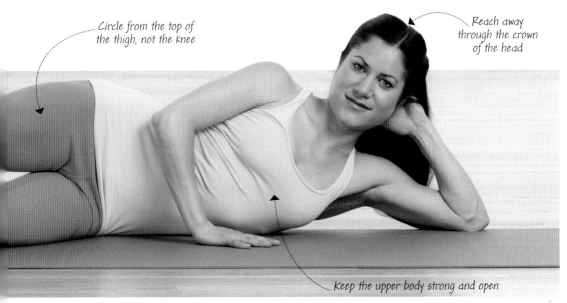

Circle from the top of the thigh, not the knee

Reach away through the crown of the head

Keep the upper body strong and open

Side Kicks: Inner Thighs

Strengthen Inner Thighs • **Practice** Concentration

This exercise really targets the areas others can't reach—
toning the inner thighs. You'll feel the burn if you concentrate
on moving with perfect alignment and control.

1 Lie on your side, using the
mat to guide your alignment,
with shoulders and hips stacked.
Press your head into your hand.
Bend the top leg in and take hold
of the ankle, placing the foot flat
on the floor. Rotate the bottom leg
so that the knee is facing down.

Tip Keep the bottom leg turned
out, like a key turning in a lock.
This will focus the work on the
inner thigh.

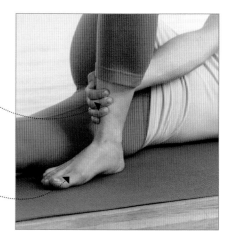

*Hold the ankle
of the top leg*

*Point the toes
toward the
bottom foot*

Leg position

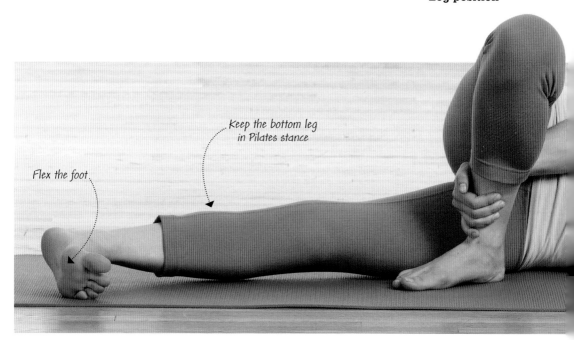

*Keep the bottom leg
in Pilates stance*

Flex the foot

2 Connect to your powerhouse and lift the left leg up as high as you can, squeezing the inner thigh. Kick up swiftly, then slowly lower. Breathe naturally throughout. Kick 10 times.

Remember Concentrate on the inner thighs doing the work and try to soften other parts of your body.

Take care...

Try not to move the upper body as the thighbone lifts. Lengthen out through the neck and keep the upper body strong and stable.

Don't lift your leg too high. Take it as far as you can without slumping the waist. Keep the rib cage lifted.

Feel the inner thigh muscle working

Keep your eyes focused forward

Press out through the heel

Press the head into the hand, reaching out through the crown of the head

Open Leg Rocker Preparation

Strengthen Stomach • **Practice** Centering

Practice this to prepare for Open Leg Rocker (see pp.156–157). It requires the harmony of all Pilates principles: smooth coordination with the breath; flowing movements; a strong, stable center; and control.

1 Sit tall and draw the legs in toward your chest, holding them around the ankles. Balance, tipping back off the sit bones. Keep the spine long, eyes focused forward, and lift through the crown of the head. Draw the belly in strongly and lengthen the neck, shoulders soft and down.

Tip Try to find a serene balance, without holding tension anywhere in the body.

Hands hold around the ankles

Position of hands

Shoulders relaxed and open

Keep knees shoulder-width apart

Feet together, softly pointed

Keep the spine long

... Lift the crown
of the head

Keep legs
shoulder-
width apart

2 Breathe in as you lengthen both legs toward the ceiling, as straight as you can. Keep the upper body open. Breathe out and bend the knees, as for step 1. Repeat 2–3 times. Extend the legs once more and balance.

Careful! Try not to allow the tailbone to curl underneath you. Press the legs into the hands to help you to balance.

Activate the
backs of the legs

Connect shoulders
into the back

The arms
stay strong
and straight

Keep the
legs long
and steady

Keep the spine
long and
supported

3 Breathe out and draw the legs together, squeezing your inner thighs, then open again. Stay long in the spine throughout and keep it supported. Bend the knees to return to the position shown in step 1. Repeat the sequence another 2–3 times.

Tip Concentrate on your balance, focusing on a point in front of you, and stay steady as you hold the legs strong.

Make it easier

Hold the legs around the knees instead, if you are finding it hard to maintain balance. Then, softly bend the knees.

Neck is
long

Hold behind
the knees

Take care...

Don't let the upper body collapse as you lengthen the legs. Use your powerhouse, abdominals, and the muscles between your shoulder blades to keep the body strong and open.

Teaser Preparation

Strengthen Stomach and Inner Thighs • **Practice** Control

This exercise builds up the strength for the Teaser (see pp.170–175) by breaking it down, precisely and slowly strengthening the deep abdominals and inner thighs.

1 Lie on your back, with feet flat on the floor. Float the arms above and behind you. Keep the rib cage heavy on the mat, and abdominals flat.

Careful! Keep the rib cage heavy as you reach the arms above you, to prevent the back from arching.

Squeeze the legs together.

Keep the feet heavy and grounded

Reach the arms and palms up

2 Breathe out to float the arms above the head and forward, nod the chin toward the chest, and curl the spine off the mat. Scoop the belly in.

Imagine Think of your spine as a feather, being lifted lightly from the floor without strain.

Lengthen the head at the end of the spine

Press the palms forward

Press the feet into the mat

3 Keep your C-curve until you find your tailbone, then open the chest and straighten the back. Breathe in to lengthen the spine. Breathe out and roll down slowly, bone by bone, to the start. Repeat 3 times.

Why? By moving on the out breath, the abdominal muscles can be more deeply recruited as you expel air from the lungs.

Keep the neck long and relaxed

Reach the arms above the knees

Keep the knees squeezed together

Keep the waist long and lifted

Feet evenly released into the floor

Reach away with the leg

More of a challenge

To make it harder, when you reach the top, lengthen one leg away, squeezing the knees together and keeping the spine long. Hold this position for 1 or 2 breaths, making sure you don't curl the tail underneath you or collapse the chest. Float the foot down and repeat with the other leg. Then roll down as before and repeat 3 times.

Teaser with Twist

Strengthen Stomach • **Practice** Centering

This exercise is a very effective waist whittler. It demands
a lot of strength from your waist. You'll need rock-solid
abdominals and great core control for this.

Reach the arms
in parallel to
the leg

Point the
foot softly

1 Sit tall, with your legs
connected. Reach your arms
above the knees. Lengthen the
right leg, keeping the knees
squeezed together. Breathe
in to lengthen the spine as you
reach the leg away to avoid
collapsing. Scoop the belly.

Imagine Try to feel as if you are
being lifted toward the ceiling.

Keep the leg
straight

Keep the shoulders
soft into the back

Keep the eyes focused
toward the leg

Scoop the
belly deeply

Reach the leg away
with energy

Curl down, keeping
a strong, lifted belly

2 Breathe out, deepen the
abdominals, and curl the
spine down, rolling bone by bone,
to the shoulder blades. Breathe in.
Keep your eyes focused forward.

Remember Think about lift and
length. Try to prevent your body
from collapsing, and stay strong.

Relax the shoulders away from the ears

Reach the arms in line with the shoulders

3 Breathe out and curl up, then twist the body across the extended leg. Return to center as you breathe in. Repeat 3 times, twisting to each side.

Help! The abdominals will want to bunch as you twist. Keep scooping deeply to really connect to the powerhouse.

Keep the leg straight

Twist from the waist

Squeeze the inner thighs

What not to do

Don't let the leg bend

Take care...

Don't twist from the shoulders; twist from the waist. Feel the twist deeply in the obliques, right under the rib cage.

Don't let the chest collapse. Keep the shoulders open and square as you move the torso. Keep thinking of your box.

Don't lower or bend the extended leg. Keep reaching out through this leg. Stay strong in the inner thighs and the powerhouse.

Swimming

Strengthen Upper Back and Buttocks
Practice Flowing Movement

A fast-moving exercise that tones the back and buttocks and shows how Pilates strengthens the body, by focusing on symmetrical movement. Concentrate on working each side evenly, with length.

1 Lie face down. Engage your center deeply as you lengthen the arms and legs away and up. The arms are at shoulder height and the legs in Pilates stance.

Imagine Think about working under water: feel the resistance and the flow of the body against the water.

Keep the arms and fingertips long

Reach the legs actively away

Keep the belly strong to protect the lower back

Point the feet softly

Keep the legs straight, in Pilates stance

2 Extend the spine so your gaze is focused forward. Reach your right arm and left leg away. Keep the belly strong.

Careful! Keep the lower spine long, hips open, and belly working throughout to protect the lower back.

Focus the eyes forward

Lengthen and support the lower spine

3 Pick up the pace as you move the opposite arms and legs up and down in a swimming motion. Breathe in for 5 counts, then out for 5. Stay strong. Continue for up to 30 counts. Then relax back down.

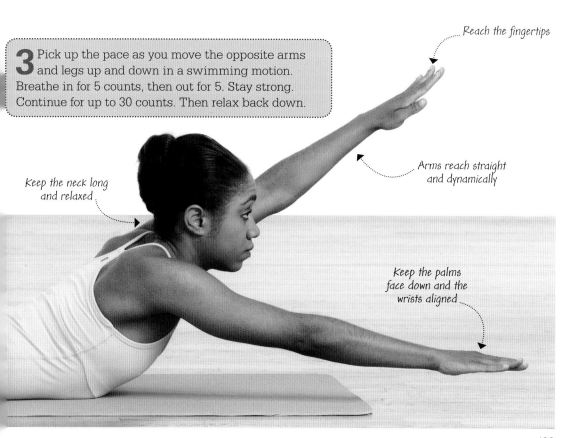

Reach the fingertips

Arms reach straight and dynamically

Keep the neck long and relaxed

Keep the palms face down and the wrists aligned

Leg Swings: Front

Strengthen Core and Buttocks • **Practice** Precision

This exercise teaches you to move freely, almost like you did when you were a child. It boosts your heart rate, challenges your balance, and checks your posture.

Fold the arms at shoulder height

Keep the shoulders soft and down

Lift the abdominals

Keep the ribs soft

Swing the knee up to your chest

Keep the pelvis square

Maintain the turnout of the supporting leg

Turn out the legs in Pilates stance

Press down into the supporting foot

1 Stand tall, squeezing the legs in Pilates stance, with your arms crossed in front. Connect to your powerhouse, with shoulders relaxed and neck long. Deeply draw the abdominals in and up toward the spine.

2 Breathe out and swing the right knee in toward your chest. Keep the spine long, and avoid tucking in the pelvis. Place the foot down swiftly as you breathe in. Switch legs. Repeat, to do 10 on each side.

Leg Swings: Side

Strengthen Hips • **Practice** Control

This exercise is wonderful if you suffer from tight hips. Strong core and balance is needed to ensure no movement ricochets through the rest of the body.

1 Stand tall in Pilates stance. Keep the arms out at shoulder height, palms facing downward. Lengthen your neck. Connect to your powerhouse and soften the shoulders. Breathe in to prepare.

Tip Keep the torso long and stable. Make sure the shoulders stay level. It helps to practice this in front of a mirror.

Keep the arms in your peripheral vision

Keep the ribs soft into the front of your body

Work the inner thighs and buttocks throughout

Spread the feet in Pilates stance

Swing the knee up toward the elbow

Keep the arms long and at shoulder height

The hips stay square

Point the foot

2 As you breathe out, kick your right knee up and out to the side, toward the elbow. Lower the leg. Alternate the legs, increasing the energy of the movement each time. Maintain a strong and stable center.

Imagine Feel the crown of your head being pulled up toward the ceiling as you swing the leg.

15-Minute Sequence

1 **Ten by Ten**
pp.92–93

2 **Half Roll Up**
pp.94–95

5 **Single Leg Stretch 2**
p.100

6 **Double Leg Stretch 2**
pp.102–103

9 **Side Kicks: Scissors**
pp.116–117

10 **Teaser Preparation**
pp.124–125

3 Rolling Like a Ball 2
pp.98–99

4 Mini Bridge
p.96

7 Neck Roll
pp.106–107

8 Side Kicks: Front 2
pp.114–115

11 Swimming
pp.128–129

12
Leg Swings:
Front
p.130

30-Minute Sequence

1 Ten by Ten
pp.92–9

2 Half Roll Up
pp.94–95

3 Rolling Like
a Ball 2
pp.98–99

7 Mini Bridge
p.96

8 Single Leg Stretch 2
p.100

9 Double Leg Stretch 2
pp.102–103

13 Neck Roll
pp.106–107

14 Spine Stretch
Forward 2
pp.104–105

15 Neck Pull
pp.112–113

19

**Magic Circle:
Pliés**
p.110

4 Side Kicks:
Front 2
pp.114–115

5 Side Kicks:
Scissors
pp.116–117

6 Side Kicks:
Circles
pp.118–119

10 Open Leg Rocker
Preparation
pp.122–123

11 Teaser Preparation
pp.124–125

12 Swimming
pp.128–129

16 Leg Swings:
Front
p.130

17 Leg
Swings:
Side
p.131

18 Magic Circle:
Inner Thighs
and Arms
p.111

45-Minute Sequence

1 **Ten by Ten**
pp.92–93

2 **Half Roll Up**
pp.94–95

3 **Rolling Like a Ball 2**
pp.98–99

7 **Mini Bridge**
p.96

8 **Single Leg Stretch 2**
p.100

9 **Single Straight Leg Stretch**
p.101

13 **Double Leg Stretch 2**
pp.102–103

14 **Neck Roll**
pp.106–107

15 **Spine Stretch Forward 2**
pp.104–105

19 **Neck Pull**
pp.112–113

20 **Side Kicks: Front 2**
pp.114–115

21 **Side Kicks: Scissors**
pp.116–117

4 Side Kicks: Circles
pp.118–119

5 Side Kicks: Inner Thighs
pp.120–121

6 Open Leg Rocker Preparation
pp.122–123

10 Teaser Preparation
pp.124–125

11 Letter T
p.97

12 Swimming
pp.128–129

16 Leg Swings: Front
p.130

17 Leg Swings: Side
p.131

18 Magic Circle: Chest and Overhead
p.108

22 Magic Circle: Pumping
p.109

23 Magic Circle: Inner Thighs and Arms
p.111

24 Magic Circle: Pliés
p.110

Assess your progress

How did you progress over the last six weeks? Go back and check your baselines (see pp.90–91). How do you feel compared to the first time you performed the exercises? Did you notice an improvement? If so, well done! Keep at it!

Common problems

Have you made less progress than you had hoped? Don't be discouraged. Pilates at this stage presents an even greater challenge: The more you understand, the more you will realize there is to understand. You should by now be concentrating on all the various techniques and principles while you exercise, so you will have more body awareness and will be more aware of any weaknesses. This is a good thing, so don't worry or allow your enthusiasm to flag. Remember Pilates is all about the detail—if you are struggling, always revisit the basics and the principles, and the answers may be found there. Here are some common problems that you might face at this stage.

"It's hard to coordinate my breathing to the movement."

As long as you're breathing rather than holding your breath, you're halfway there. The breathing pattern is one of the most common things that people struggle with, so you're not alone. At this stage, the exercises become more dynamic and the need for controlled, coordinated breathing is greater. Memorize the exercise's breathing pattern: then, you will know exactly what you should be doing and won't lose focus during the exercise. Concentrate solely on breathing for a few workouts: you will begin to find it makes sense in your body and with the movement. Above all, never hold your breath as you move, because it will make you tense.

"I find the side-lying exercises really difficult on one side."

This is very common: Pilates will highlight any imbalances that we have in the muscles and skeleton. Often, we favor one side of the body more than the other in daily movement, which causes it to become stronger. If you find the exercises on one side significantly harder and your body less stable, don't give up. Perform more repetitions on this side to try to strengthen it and balance the body.

"I simply can't do a particular exercise."

Keep practicing; it will come. Break the exercise down and practice each section individually to work out which part is causing you trouble. Repeat this movement over and over, to train both your body and mind. Being determined will reap rewards. If a particular exercise is causing you pain or aggravating a part of the body, however, it is probably best to avoid the exercise, or substitute another one for it. For example, if your lower back is aggravated by a rolling exercise, omit it or replace it with one from the first chapter (see pp.26–87) until you feel stronger and more controlled, and able to tackle it again.

Assess your achievement

Didn't achieve your goals? Don't lose your inspiration as you move on to the final section of the book (see pp.140–185). Celebrate every achievement as you practice, for example being able to roll your spine smoothly into a C-curve, or to straighten your leg slightly farther than before. Small achievements build up—soon you'll be setting yourself new goals.

Challenging exercises

Here is a plan to help you during your workouts over the next six weeks. At the end of the six weeks, look back over these goals and assess how you have progressed.

Goal: Control
Teaser with Twist (see pp.126–127)

Work on twisting smoothly, remaining strong and lifted

Goal: Centering
Double Leg Stretch 2
(see pp.102–103)

Work on flowing movement from a strong core, keeping the spine strong and supported

Goal: Flexibility
Single Straight Leg Stretch
(see p.101)

Work on straightening each leg directly to the ceiling and keeping it long

Goal: Strength
Ten by Ten (see pp.92–93),
Half Roll Up (see pp.94–95),
Teaser Preparation (see pp.124–125)

Work on staying strong through each exercise, flowing each one to the next without a break

Goal: Flowing Movement
Swimming (see pp.128–129)

Work on moving the limbs smoothly from a relaxed torso, without stopping and starting

3
Take It Further

The exercises in this chapter require you to have mastered all of the earlier exercises as well as to understand and be able to put in to practice the fundamental principles of Pilates. Perform each of these final, more demanding exercises precisely, fluidly, and purposefully, only moving on to the sequences once you are fully confident with your ability to perform each individual exercise. Once you have completed the course in this book, you should be well-equipped to continue practicing Pilates, and will reap the benefits of a strong, supple, and balanced body.

Plan Your Program

We're nearly at the end of the program! You should be really seeing the results by now, with sculpted limbs, a supple spine, and a honed midriff, not to mention feeling brighter and clearer as you breathe more easily and stand taller.

Planning the next step

I hope your progress so far has inspired you to continue with just as much enthusiasm as you possessed at the start. Now we want to take the next challenge into the more advanced Pilates exercises on the mat, working our bodies even harder. Keep focusing on the detail and you will find that these dynamic exercises offer an amazing sense of achievement for your body. We will continue to use broadly the same goals as for the first two stages of the program, so that we have a good idea of how far we have come when we reach the end.

Build On It Exercise Program

Use this program to set yourself goals and assess your progress over the next six weeks. Summaries of the sequences are on pp.178–183. Each week, when you work out, follow the sequences in this program for the first few times. After that, you could mix exercises in from the rest of the section—but take care to substitute any with an exercise that trains the same area of the body, so your workout is balanced. Remember to act as your own coach and perform every movement to the best of your ability.

Week 1: Focus on Alignment
Baseline: The original photographs you took at the start of the Start Simple Exercise Programme (see pp.28–29).
• **Day 1:** 30-minute sequence, check centering, control

• **Day 2:** 15-minute sequence, check lengthening, coordination
• **Day 3:** 45-minute sequence, check precision, flowing movement
• **Day 4:** 30-minute sequence, check stability, breathing
Goal: Take new photos after six weeks to see how much closer you are to your ideal alignment.

Week 2: Focus on Control
Baseline: Perform the Corkscrew (see pp.160–161). Are you moving smoothly through the hips, or stiffly and jerkily? Can you hold the legs together and connect to your powerhouse throughout? Are the legs moving in a circle or more of a square?
• **Day 1:** 45-minute sequence, check centering, alignment
• **Day 2:** 30-minute sequence, check concentration, precision, scoop
• **Day 3:** 45-minute sequence, check precision, breathing, Pilates box
• **Day 4:** 15-minute sequence, check flowing movement, stability
Goal: Do the exercise with control, precision, and fluidity, remembering powerhouse, scooping, and lengthening.

Week 3: Focus on Centering

Baseline: perform Scissors (see pp.168–169). Is the back arched? Is the spine still and supported as you move the legs?

- **Day 1:** 30-minute sequence, check box, alignment, flowing movement
- **Day 2:** 30-minute sequence, check stability, precision, lengthening
- **Day 3:** 45-minute sequence, check precision, control, breathing
- **Day 4:** 30-minute sequence, check control, alignment

Goal: Aim for no unwanted movement of the spine as you lengthen the limbs away, smoothly and in control.

Week 4: Focus on Flexibility

Baseline: perform Open Leg Rocker (see pp.156–157). Are you able to keep both legs straight up to the ceiling? Does your spine roll evenly on the floor?

- **Day 1:** 30-minute sequence, check precision, control, alignment
- **Day 2:** 30-minute sequence, check breathing, scoop, stability
- **Day 3:** 45-minute sequence, check scoop, powerhouse, coordination
- **Day 4:** 15-minute sequence, check control, concentration

Goal: Keep the legs straight and lengthened, and roll the spine through each vertebra evenly.

Week 5: Focus on Strength

Baseline: Try performing Teaser 1, Teaser 2, and Teaser 3 (see pp.170–175) without a break. On a scale of 1 to 10, how hard was each exercise and the sequence?

- **Day 1:** 45-minute sequence, check centering, control, coordination
- **Day 2:** 30-minute sequence, check scoop, alignment, concentration
- **Day 3:** 15-minute sequence, check alignment, coordination, flowing movement
- **Day 4:** 45-minute sequence, check control, precision, powerhouse

Goal: When you do the sequence again, it should feel easier.

Week 6: Focus on Flowing Movement

Baseline: Perform Rocking (see pp.176–177). Does the movement feel fluid and controlled or jerky and broken? Can you rock smoothly without stopping and starting?

- **Day 1:** 30-minute sequence, check centering, breathing, coordination
- **Day 2:** 45-minute sequence, check stability, control, Pilates box
- **Day 3:** 15-minute sequence, check alignment, lengthening, coordination
- **Day 4:** 45-minute sequence, check precision, centering, breathing

Goal: Make the movement smoother as you engage your powerhouse to begin rocking, without any wobbling or stopping.

Check your new baseline for each area of the body before you begin this exercise program and make a note of how it feels to do each movement. Then, at the end of the six weeks, assess yourself, according to the goals given here, to see how far you have gone toward achieving your targets. Enjoy the next six weeks!

The Hundred

Strengthen Stomach • **Practice** Breathing

Joe Pilates's original "classic" version of The Hundred requires
deep abdominal strength, control, and precision. It warms up
the body, and fires up the powerhouse.

1 Lie on your mat, shoulders open, arms relaxed by your sides, and legs reaching away, connected in the Pilates stance. Lift into your powerhouse, squeeze the legs, and breathe in to prepare.

Squeeze the legs in Pilates stance

Keep the feet softly pointed

Keep the neck long and relaxed

Press the arms down by your sides

Keep the collarbones wide

Connect the shoulders into the body

Take care...

Don't tilt your head back. Keep your neck long and eyes forward. Use your belly to curl up more, rather than allowing the neck to drop back.

Don't let your arms become floppy. Your arms should pump from the shoulder joint freely, pressing out through the palms.

2 Breathe out, scoop your belly, and curl the head and shoulders off the mat, reaching your arms forward with energy. Keep the neck long, and shoulders away from your ears. Simultaneously, lift your legs away, keeping them as close to the floor as you can control.

Careful! If you feel a strain in the neck or lower back, bring the legs slightly higher and deepen your abdominal connection.

Reach the arms dynamically away

Turn the legs out from the hips

Keep the neck long and free from tension

3 Breathe in and pump the arms dynamically for a count of 5. Breathe out and pump for another count of 5. Give a long, even exhalation as you pump, not a staccato breath. Suspend the head and legs easily in space as you pump smoothly. Repeat this pattern until you reach 100 pumps. Pause to lengthen the body, then release down with control.

Imagine Think of lightness. It should look effortless, not strained.

Squeeze the inner thighs

Pump the arms up and down with your breaths

Keep the feet 4–6in (10–15cm) away from the floor

145

Roll Over

Strengthen Stomach, Thighs, Buttocks, and Arms
Practice Concentration

A massage for the spine, this exercise works the abdominals to
peel the spine smoothly from the mat. You need control and a
strong core to prevent momentum from carrying the legs over.

1 Lie on your mat. Engage your center. Float your
legs into the chest, then extend them up to the
ceiling. Rotate your legs into the Pilates stance,
engaging the buttock and thigh muscles.

Remember Squeeze the legs together from the inner
thighs to the heels. Feel the buttocks wrapping
around, connecting the legs tightly.

Point the toes softly

Keep the legs straight up above the hip joints

Release the arms into the floor

Squeeze the buttocks

Keep the legs in line with the floor, and no lower

2 Breathe out; curl the spine bone by bone to lift the
hips, sending the legs over the head, parallel with
the floor. Work the arms to support your body weight.

Why? The legs are active, so you are
aware of the whole body contributing
to the dynamics of the movement.

Lift your hips away from the rib cage.

Press the arms into the mat, keeping palms long

3 Breathe in and flex the feet. Breathe out and lower down with control, bone by bone. Keep the legs straight and reaching away.

Imagine Think of having spines on your back like those on a dinosaur's back. Each of these must lock into the floor individually as your torso rolls down.

Press out through the heels of your flexed feet

Keep the legs long and straight

Maintain strong thighs

Roll down evenly through the spine

4 When you reach your tailbone, lengthen your legs toward the floor, with the belly strong and feet flexed. Close your legs into the Pilates stance, then use the strength of your belly to pick them up and roll over again. Repeat 5 times.

Careful! The legs tend to bend and become limp. Keep them active, lifted, and strong.

The heels press up

Release the tailbone down slowly

Keep the neck relaxed and long

Press the palms into the mat

Climb a Tree

Strengthen Stomach • **Practice** Precision

This exercise clearly highlights any imbalances you have in your body. It requires great control and strength—with one leg in the air there is no way you can cheat!

1 Sit tall, left leg reaching away and right leg bent in toward you. Lengthen the right leg toward the ceiling, then bend it again. Repeat 3 times.

Remember Draw the belly in tight, waist long and chest open.

Keep the chest open

Keep the leg bent

Keep the supporting leg heavy and active

Keep the spine long and lifted

Reach the leg strong and straight

Keep the hands around the ankle

Connect the shoulders into the back

2 On the third reach, walk your hands up the leg to take hold of the ankle. Keep strong and lifted in the waist.

Tip Lift the body higher as if you are opening your chest toward your foot.

Keep the lower spine protected

The supporting leg stays heavy and long

Keep the leg straight, foot softly pointed

3 Breathe in. Lengthen the right leg to the ceiling as you curl the spine down, walking your hands down your leg. Go as far as your shoulder blades, keeping the eyes focused toward the knee.

Careful! Keep the movement slow. Don't let your body drop.

Point the foot softly

Reach the leg straight to the ceiling

Lift through the crown of the head

Keep the hands behind the thigh

Reach through the supporting foot

Connect the shoulders into the back

Keep the hands around the ankle

Keep the head lengthened at the end of the spine

4 Breathe out and climb back up the leg with your hands. Try to straighten the leg as much as you can. Repeat twice; switch legs.

Help! If one side feels more difficult, use your abs to control it.

Keep the elbows wide

Stay heavy and grounded with the supporting leg

Curl up the spine

Point the toes

Footwork 1

Strengthen Thighs and Buttocks • **Practice** Concentration

This standing exercise works your muscles against gravity in a slightly unusual way. You need balance and focus to perform this correctly. Toned buttocks and thighs will be your reward!

Keep the elbows wide

Keep the waist long

Lift the belly

Turn the feet out, keeping the heels connected

Press the hands behind the head

Lift the crown of the head

Bend the knees over the toes

Feel the toe joints stretching

1 Stand tall, in Pilates stance. Release your shoulders into your back and lengthen the waist. Lift into your center. Place your hands behind your head, keeping the elbows wide.

Remember Keep lifting through the crown of the head throughout.

2 Breathe in, bend the knees, and lower the tailbone directly to the floor. The heels rise. At the bottom, press the heels down and rise back to standing. Repeat 6 times, breathing in to lower and breathing out to lift.

Careful! If you have knee problems, avoid this exercise.

Footwork 2

Strengthen Buttocks • **Practice** Precision

This is a simple exercise, but it requires control and precision.
It will give great toning results if performed correctly. Think
about your alignment and strong core throughout.

Keep the arms at chest height

Keep the waist long

Scoop the abdominals in and up

Keep the legs parallel

Keep the feet evenly grounded

Lift the crown of the head toward the ceiling

Keep the arms level with the chest

Keep the rib cage soft

Work the buttocks

Keep the knees directly over the toes

1 Stand tall, with the legs hip-width apart and in parallel. Keep the arms crossed in front of your chest and shoulders released and away from the ears. Draw the belly in toward the spine.

Remember Think about your box. Keep it long and square.

2 Bend your knees as low as you can while keeping your balance. Press yourself up, using your center. Repeat 6 times. Breathe in to lower and breathe out to rise back up.

Imagine As you bend, think of your core like a dimmer switch, turning up its engagement to support the movement.

Double Straight Leg Stretch

Strengthen Stomach • **Practice** Control

This exercise hones the mid-section of the body well,
tightening the waist and working on the six-pack.
It also develops your strength and stamina.

Keep the knees
pointed at the ceiling

Keep the feet
parallel with
the floor

Keep the
head heavy

1 Lie centrally on the mat, with
legs in toward the chest. Keep
the thighs soft and relaxed in
their sockets. Place your hands
behind your head, elbows wide
and open, and breathe in to
lengthen the spine.

Keep the feet
softly pointed

Squeeze the
legs together

Constantly scoop
in the belly

2 Breathe out and curl the upper
body off the mat, extending
the legs toward the ceiling and
squeezing them together in the
Pilates stance. Engage the
buttocks and thighs and softly
point the feet. Look in toward
your navel and scoop the belly.

Help! If this is tough on your
thighs and you feel them gripping,
bend the knees slightly.

3 Breathe in and lower the legs down toward the mat, only as far as you can control the movement. Breathe out and draw them back slowly, wrapping the buttock muscles around. Keep your upper body strong and still. Repeat 8 times.

Tip Focus on your center, keeping the core strong as you lengthen the legs away.

Squeeze the heels

Keep the legs straight and strong

Don't allow the head to drop back

Keep the elbows in your peripheral vision

Feel the muscles of the backs of the legs

Keep the curl high

Keep the rib cage heavy

153

Criss-cross

Strengthen Stomach and Waist • **Practice** Flowing Movement

This exercise is a waist cincher like no other. Focus on moving precisely, with flow. When you start to tire toward the end, keep moving with control and you will see dramatic results.

1 Start by doing the Double Straight Leg Stretch (see pp.152–53). Keep your hands behind your head and fold the knees in. Breathe in and curl up, press one leg away, and twist the spine toward the bent leg. Keep the elbows wide and the waist long. Pause.

Bend the knee in

Look toward the elbow

Press the leg in line with the body

2 Breathe out, switch legs, and rotate to the opposite knee. Keep the abdominals sinking toward the spine. Repeat 6 times on each side; as you twist from side to side, stay curled up. Then relax down.

Bring the knee in toward you

Press the leg away with energy

Keep the head heavy in the hands

Spine Stretch Forward 3

Strengthen Upper Back and Stomach • **Practice** Breathing

This exercise combines Spine Stretch Forward 1 (see p.66)
and 2 (see pp.104–105), and involves moving through the spine with
control, using the breath, and working the abs to stretch the spine.

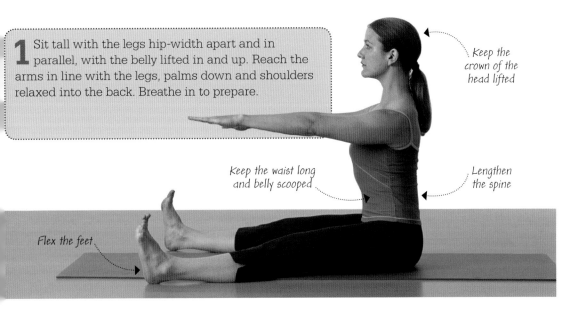

1 Sit tall with the legs hip-width apart and in parallel, with the belly lifted in and up. Reach the arms in line with the legs, palms down and shoulders relaxed into the back. Breathe in to prepare.

Keep the crown of the head lifted

Keep the waist long and belly scooped

Lengthen the spine

Flex the feet

2 Breathe out and roll the spine forward in a C-curve, reaching the arms above and parallel to the legs. Breathe in to deepen the stretch. Breathe out to roll back up, bone by bone, growing taller as you re-stack.

Lengthen the neck

Keep the shoulders connected into the back

Pull the toes back toward you

Keep the belly scooping up and back

Open Leg Rocker

Strengthen Stomach • **Practice** Control

Rhythm, balance, flexibility, core strength, and control are all
required here. The rolling should appear smooth and effortless,
but underneath there needs to be strict control and precision.

Open legs to
shoulder-width

Press the
legs into
the hands

Keep spine
straight and
lengthened

1 Sit on your mat with room
to roll back. Float the legs to
the ceiling, just wider than the
shoulders, holding on around
the ankles. Open your chest and
connect your shoulders into your
back. Connect deeply to your
center. Breathe in to prepare.

Imagine Think of your body as
a perfect "V" shape.

Keep legs straight
and active

Reach the tailbone
toward the ceiling

Keep arms straight
and strong

2 Breathe out and, maintaining
the same position, curl your
tailbone under and allow yourself
to rock back as far as your
shoulder blades. Nod the chin to
the chest and look at your center.

Remember Keep the "V" shape
as you rock back. Reach the
thighbones away from your center.

3 Breathe in, and pause at the bottom of the movement. Then breathe out and roll back up, activating the backs of the thighs. Balance at the top, with the chest open. Repeat up to 8 times. To finish, float your feet down.

Imagine Think of your spine as a wheel rolling on a track, rolling back and forth along exactly the same section evenly.

Take care...

Avoid tipping the head back. Let the movement come from the tilting of the hips, and then smoothly roll onto the spine. The head stays aligned at the end of the spine.

Don't hunch the shoulders. Doing this drags the body toward the legs. Keep the arms long and light, the shoulders connected down and back. The limbs stay exactly in position as the spine rocks the body.

Feet softly pointed

Keep the head in line with the spine

Keep the legs straight

Engage the buttocks

Keep the spine central on your mat

Seal

Strengthen Back and Stomach • **Practice** Concentration

This exercise evokes the playful movement of childhood, while also toning the abdominals and massaging the spine. It is a great challenge for your core strength, balance, and coordination.

1 Sit tall on your mat. Thread your hands through your legs to grab hold of the outsides of your ankles. Tilt your hips to lift your feet from the mat. Balance momentarily, scooping in your belly. Clap the insides of the feet together 3 times, imitating a seal. Lengthen the spine and draw in the belly.

Help! Practice this without the foot claps at first if it is too hard to coordinate the movement.

Grasp the outsides of the ankles

Keep the hips open

Keep the knees shoulder-width apart

Keep your head off the floor

Roll the lower spine off the mat

2 Breathe in and roll back smoothly, as far as the shoulder blades. Keep your chin tucked into your chest to make sure your head doesn't roll back. The tailbone reaches up toward the ceiling. Pause here momentarily and clap the feet 3 times once more.

3 Breathe out and deepen your powerhouse connection to roll back to the start position. Clap the feet as you balance, then roll back again smoothly. Repeat up to 10 times, breathing in to roll back and out to roll forward. The movement is swift and fluid.

Tip Use your breath. The forceful exhalation helps you to connect to the abdominals and to muster the power to roll forward with control.

Keep the head aligned with the spine

Knees stay open

Keep the feet together

Keep the spine in a C-curve

Take care...

Don't drop your head back when initiating the roll. The head should nod toward the chest throughout the movement, keeping the neck long.

Don't straighten the back at the top of the movement. Keep the C-curve active throughout; you should feel as if you could roll continuously.

Corkscrew

Strengthen Stomach, Inner Thighs, and Buttocks
Practice Centering

Corkscrew requires strong control and a deep connection to
your powerhouse. You need to move smoothly with no tension
or strain as the abdominals take the weight of the legs.

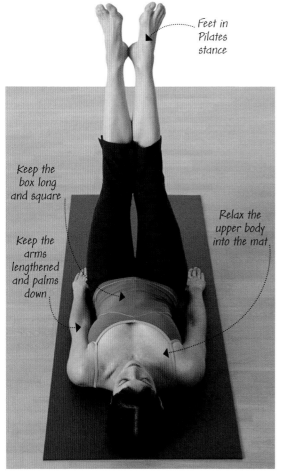

Feet in
Pilates
stance

Keep the
box long
and square

Keep the
arms
lengthened
and palms
down

Relax the
upper body
into the mat

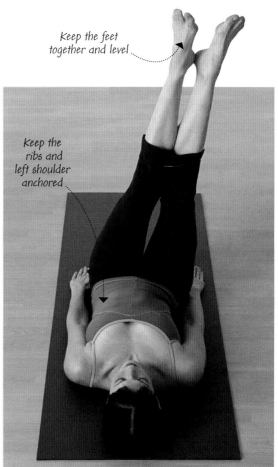

Keep the feet
together and level

Keep the
ribs and
left shoulder
anchored

1 Lie flat on the mat, legs stretched directly
up above your hips. Imagine a clock face
above you, with your legs pointing straight
up to twelve o'clock. Soften the knees if you
feel the thighs are gripping.

2 Breathe in and squeeze the legs together
as you tilt the pelvis to rock across to your
right and bring the legs to one o'clock. Keep
the torso heavy. Move only the legs—the hips
and ribs should not lift.

Make it easier

Place your hands on the mat to brace the lower back and press the elbows down to the mat. Follow the exercise. If you still have back pain while doing this exercise, stop.

Take care...

Make sure you keep your legs and feet glued together throughout. Feel the movement coming from the tops of the thighbones and pelvis.

Don't rock the shoulders or ribs. To isolate the movement in the hips, connect to your center and concentrate on controlling the movement.

Maintain your Pilates stance

Keep the belly strong and flat

Keep the palms relaxed and heavy

Keep the legs together throughout

Keep rib cage heavy and grounded

3 Circle the legs forward and down to six o'clock, lowering them as they go. Keep the abdominals strongly scooped as you release the legs forward. Feel the lower back supported by the abdominals.

4 Circle the legs across and up to eleven o'clock, at your left. Breathe out to complete the circle and take the legs back to twelve o'clock. Repeat the whole circle, but in the opposite direction. Then repeat 2–3 sets.

Saw

Strengthen Waist and Back • **Practice** Breathing

Joe Pilates wanted us to "wring all the air out of the lungs" as
you would wring water from a wet cloth. Here, bending the
spine on the out breath facilitates this sensation.

Lengthen the palms, keep the fingers active and long

Lift the belly in and up

Reach the legs away

1 Sit tall, legs about shoulder-width apart, feet flexed. Float your arms out to the side, just within your peripheral vision, palms facing down, fingers long. Connect to your center, lift the waist, and pull in the abdominals.

Tip Your spine is lifting and lengthening up and away from your pelvis. Your legs are long and active.

Reach the right arm actively back, as if someone is pulling it

Take care...

Your legs shouldn't move with the twist. The twist should come from the ribs, not from the hips, so the pelvis should remain square. Check that your feet aren't moving as you twist, and keep the sit bones bolted into the floor.

Don't allow the knees to roll in. Keep the feet and knees parallel with the ceiling to make sure you are in good alignment.

Keep the pelvis square

Arms stay in line with the shoulders

Align the wrists with the arms

Keep the waist long

Press the legs away

2 Breathe in as you twist to the right, imagining the spine growing taller as you twist. Keep the left hip anchored and square. Press out through the heels.

Imagine Think of your rib cage as a ball twisting around a pole connected to the ceiling. Grow taller as you twist.

Sit tall on the sit bones

3 Breathe out and curl the spine forward, reaching the left hand to the outside of the right foot. Curl deeper. Breathe in to re-stack to your center, then twist to the left. Repeat 3 times on either side.

Why? Breathing out while curling forward softens the rib cage and facilitates the movement. Your belly lifts and the air is squeezed out of the lungs as you pulse farther forward.

Twist the ribs across

Reach past your foot

Swan

Strengthen Spine, Stomach, Arms, and Legs
Practice Flow, Breath, Control, and Precision
It is a challenge to perform this exercise correctly. Build up your
strength with Swan Preparation (see p.69). Move your body as
one connected unit, with strength and flow.

1 Lie face down on your mat. Squeeze your feet
together, in parallel. Extend the spine, lifting the
chest. Reach the arms out in front, pulling the
shoulder blades down and into the back to connect.

Tip Relax and lengthen the neck and keep the chest
lifted. Lift the belly to support the spine.

Open the palms to the ceiling

Softly point the feet

Lengthen the lower back

2 Breathing naturally, begin to rock on your pelvis,
initiating a small forward and backward
movement, like a boat rocking on water. Use the
powerhouse connection to increase the rocking.

Remember The momentum comes from your
powerhouse, not from reaching with the arms or
kicking the legs.

Keep the palms open

Keep your eyes focused upward

Keep the legs connected and reaching away

Lift the chest

3 As the rocking increases, reach the legs up to the ceiling to increase the downward momentum. Drive the chest up high to send the legs downward. Repeat up to 10 times. Then counterstretch by rounding your back, bending your knees, lifting your bottom, and sitting on your heels. Fold yourself into the Child's Pose (see p.17), with arms releasing forward and chest toward your thighs. Relax the forehead downward and allow the spine to release.

Tip Focus on keeping length in the body: Reach the fingertips away from the toes and allow this extension to help you find the strength for the movement.

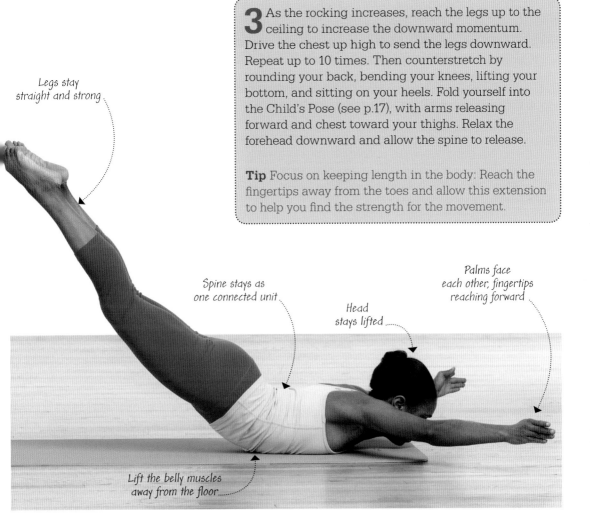

Legs stay straight and strong

Spine stays as one connected unit

Head stays lifted

Palms face each other, fingertips reaching forward

Lift the belly muscles away from the floor

Take care...

Try not to break the line of the body. Keep the body connected from your toes right to the crown of the head—your center should support the spine completely.

Don't bend your arm or legs. With the limbs straight, reach dynamically away from your center.

Make it easier

Place the hands underneath the shoulders and use them to pivot the body

Double Leg Kick

Strengthen Upper Back and Back of Thighs
Practice Concentration

This exercise opens the chest, mobilizing the upper back
and working the hamstrings. Concentrate on the muscles you
should be feeling, to ensure they are working effectively.

1 Lie face down, turn your head to the right, and rest
on your cheek. Clasp your hands behind your back,
elbows out to the sides. Relax the body into the mat,
and draw in the belly. Relax and lengthen the spine.

Place the palms as
far up the back
as they can reach

Rest on one cheek

Keep the legs
together
and parallel

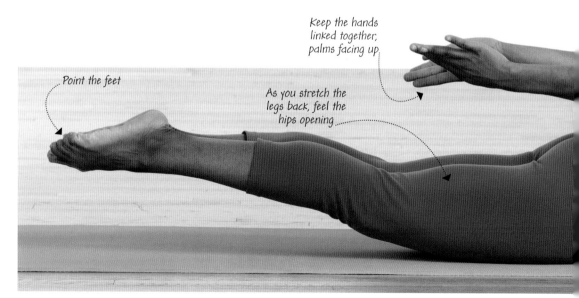

Keep the hands
linked together,
palms facing up

Point the feet

As you stretch the
legs back, feel the
hips opening

2 Breathe in and kick the heels in toward the buttocks swiftly for 3 pulses. Support the lower back by releasing your hips and pelvis heavily into the mat as you kick the legs in—try not to arch. The spine remains still and stable—make sure your belly is scooped deeply.

Take care...

Don't let the hips rise as the legs kick. Keep the front of the pelvis heavy into the mat throughout the movement.

The elbows should not be too high. Keep the elbows low and out to the side.

Keep the belly lifted

Keep the legs together as you kick

Keep the shoulders relaxed

3 Breathe out. Simultaneously reach the hands toward your buttocks as you lift straight legs. Stretch the arms back to lift the upper body. Pause here for a moment, then lower the body with control and turn the other cheek to the floor. Clasp the hands up the back and release the elbows to the sides. Repeat 3 times, alternating sides. Rest your bottom back onto your heels into the Child's Pose (see p.17) once you finish.

Feel the triceps working as you reach the arm

Keep the eyes focused forward

Take one palm into the other hand, link the thumbs, and maintain this link when the arms are outstretched

Keep the belly strong

Hand position

Scissors

Strengthen Buttocks, Stomach, and Back • **Practice** Precision

This is an incredibly demanding exercise. Protect your
shoulders and neck by maintaining a strong center
throughout, and working with length and control.

1 Lie flat on your back with your legs
extended above your hips and connected
in Pilates stance. Place your arms by your
sides and press them into the mat. Keep
the palms down, fingertips actively pressing
into the ground. Connect deeply to your
powerhouse, with waist long, belly scooped.

*Squeeze the
legs together*

*Keep the shoulders
open and heavy*

*Reach the legs
to the ceiling*

2 Scoop your belly and lift the hips,
raising your legs straight up to the
ceiling, making sure they don't tip toward
you. Place your hands behind your back for
support, with elbows flat on the floor.

Scoop the belly

*Support the
lower spine with
your hands*

*Keep the
head relaxed*

*Keep the elbows
narrow and
grounded*

3 Allow the hips to lower slightly into the hands. Pause for a moment to draw in more deeply to your center and feel balanced. Lengthen your box, scoop the belly, and feel the arms supporting your weight.

Careful! If you feel dizzy at any point, stop immediately.

Keep the feet long and reach to the ceiling

Support the pelvis with your hands

Hand position

Keep the rib cage connecting to the hips

Let the hips drop away from the body slightly

Scissor the legs evenly, taking both legs the same distance forward and back

Keep the leg straight and long, in line with the hip

4 Breathe in to scissor your legs. Breathe out and reverse. When familiar with the scissor movement, finish with a double pulse of the leg. Alternate for 5 sets. Release the hips back down slowly to finish.

Imagine Think of pressing your legs against resistance, as if stretching toffee between the legs.

Keep the neck and shoulders relaxed

Open the front of the hip as you lengthen the leg away

Teaser 1

Strengthen Stomach • **Practice** Control

This exercise concentrates on the abdominals—its pure focus
means there's no way the body can cheat. It's one of the
toughest and most effective abdominal exercises you'll ever find.

1 Lie on your back, with your knees into your chest and arms reaching behind you, in line with your ears. Keep the rib cage anchored and belly scooped. Breathe in to prepare, with the spine long and relaxed.

Point the knees to the ceiling

Engage your center

Extend the arms in line with your ears

Relax your feet

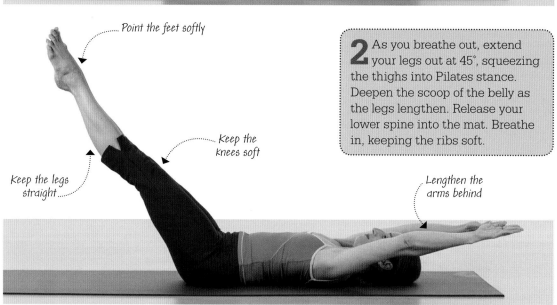

Point the feet softly

2 As you breathe out, extend your legs out at 45°, squeezing the thighs into Pilates stance. Deepen the scoop of the belly as the legs lengthen. Release your lower spine into the mat. Breathe in, keeping the ribs soft.

Keep the knees soft

Keep the legs straight

Lengthen the arms behind

3 Breathe out to curl the spine off the mat, bone by bone. Keep your shoulders relaxed as your fingers reach to the feet. Pull the belly further into the spine as you curl up toward the legs. Keep the legs high.

Careful! Make sure you control the movement upward: avoid using momentum and dragging your body up carelessly. Use the out breath and strong abdominals.

Reach the arms toward the toes

Squeeze the thighs

Keep the eyes focused forward

Keep the belly scooped

Keep the spine straight and long

4 Keep the legs perfectly still as you reach with the arms parallel to the thighs. Breathe in. Maintain the height of the legs as you slowly lower the spine down, with control. Repeat 3 times.

Help! If you need to build up your strength, practice this with your feet against a wall to become familiar with the movement.

Imagine Think of your legs suspended toward the ceiling by a crane, staying lifted as you lower the spine down to the mat. Keep the abdominals working.

Make it easier

Return to the Teaser Preparation exercises (see pp.124–125) to build up your strength for the Teaser series. Or, bend the knees and allow the legs to soften, lessening the load that your center needs to lift. Stay strong and controlled.

Walk the hands up the back of your thighs if you need to, to guide you through the movement while you build up your strength.

Bend the knees

Teaser 2

Strengthen Stomach and Spine • **Practice** Centering

Building on Teaser 1 (see pp.170–171), here we challenge the lower abdominals by lowering the legs with control while keeping the upper body lifted, firm, and stable.

1 Start by lying on your mat as for Teaser 1. If you are flowing directly from Teaser 1, move straight to Step 3 from the final position of Teaser 1.

Point the knees to the ceiling

Extend the arms in line with the ears

Keep the rib cage heavy

Relax the feet

Squeeze the feet together

Straighten the legs

Keep the belly strong

Reach the arms back

2 Deepen the scoop of the belly and extend the legs to 45°, keeping the spine stable. Continue to reach through the arms and stay anchored in the rib cage.

Imagine Your legs are light as a feather, and you are easily lifting them from your center.

3 Breathe out and use your abdominals to curl up smoothly and create a "V" shape with your body, reaching your fingers toward the toes. Draw in deeply to your powerhouse, lengthening your waist, and keeping the legs connected in Pilates stance. Find your balance.

Tip Keep the shoulders relaxed and away from the ears.

Align the head with the spine

Press the palms forward

Squeeze the legs together

Draw in the belly toward the spine

4 Keeping the upper body absolutely still, lower and lift the legs 3–5 times. Breathe in to lower and out to lift. Initiate the movement from your lower abdominals and inner thighs; try to soften the front of your legs and avoid them tensing. Slowly roll down to the start position to finish.

Help! If you find it hard to lower your legs while they are straight, practice with soft knees, keeping your toes higher than your knees.

Lift the head

Keep the arms straight

Scoop the belly even more as you lower the legs

Reach the legs away, toward the floor

Keep the spine long and supported

Teaser 3

Strengthen Stomach and Inner Thighs
Practice Flowing Movement

Teaser 1 (see pp.170–171) works the upper body and Teaser 2 (see pp.172–173) the legs. Teaser 3 combines the two movements in one workout—an unbeatable combo for flat abs and toned thighs.

1 Lie flat on your back with your arms overhead and legs outstretched in front. Bring your legs into Pilates stance: heels together, toes apart. Tighten the corset of core muscles to bring your rib cage down toward your hips and release the lower back toward the mat. Breathe in to prepare.

Squeeze the legs in Pilates stance

Draw the belly deep into the spine

Keep the toes apart

2 Breathe out, floating your arms above you. Simultaneously bring your legs up into the air, creating a "V" shape with your body. Balance on your sit bones, reaching your fingertips toward your feet.

Keep the arms parallel to the legs

Keep the chest open

Draw the belly in and up; lift the waist

Keep the legs strong and straight

3 Keeping the spine and waist long, breathe in and reach the arms above the head in line with your ears. Reach tall with the crown of your head. Stay strong and don't allow your body to crumple.

Imagine Act like you are a jack-in-the-box, springing up easily and quickly. Then slowly lower your body down.

Extend the arms in line with the ears

Softly point the feet

Scoop the belly

Curl the tailbone beneath you

Squeeze the thighs

4 Breathe out, lowering the body and legs down slowly, with control. Breathe in and momentarily pause, keeping your powerhouse active. Breathing out, spring straight back up into the "V." Repeat 5 times.

Careful! Make sure the back doesn't arch as you place the arms above the head. Keep the rib cage down and tailbone curled beneath you.

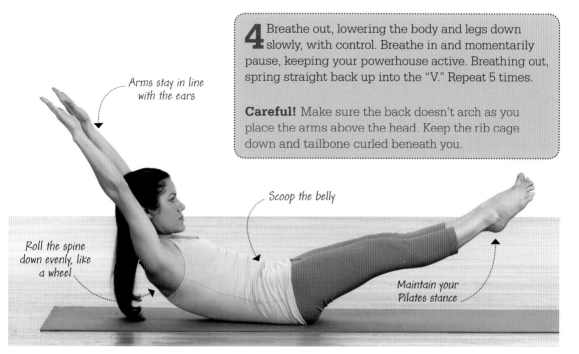

Arms stay in line with the ears

Scoop the belly

Roll the spine down evenly, like a wheel

Maintain your Pilates stance

175

Rocking

Strengthen Back • **Practice** Concentration

This exercise is the counterpose to the Teaser series, as it takes your spine into the opposite movement to stretch out and balance the body. It's a perfect way to end your abdominal workout.

1 Lie face down on your mat with your legs in parallel. Bend your knees and grab hold of your ankles. Connect your shoulders into your back and lengthen your neck. Lift your head slightly to gaze forward.

Hold around the front of the foot

Keep the neck in line with the spine

Keep the knees bent and hip-width apart

2 Extend the upper spine. Look forward. Begin to stretch the spine up into an arc by pressing the ankles into the hands. Lift the chest up and forward. Engage your buttocks and lift the thighs so your spine is arched.

Keep the arms straight

Keep the eyes focused forward

Lift the thighs off the mat

Keep the chest open and lifted

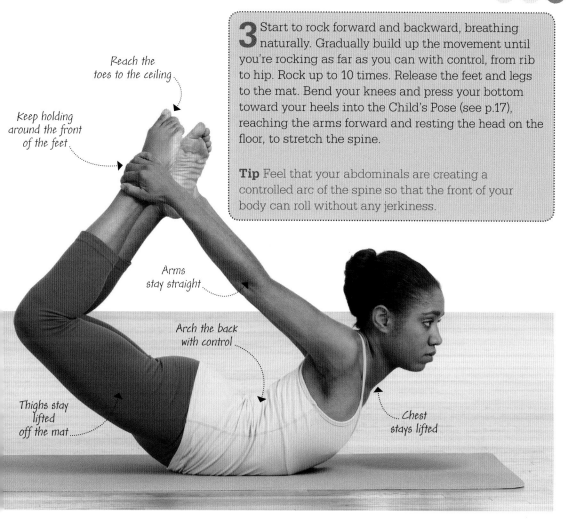

3 Start to rock forward and backward, breathing naturally. Gradually build up the movement until you're rocking as far as you can with control, from rib to hip. Rock up to 10 times. Release the feet and legs to the mat. Bend your knees and press your bottom toward your heels into the Child's Pose (see p.17), reaching the arms forward and resting the head on the floor, to stretch the spine.

Tip Feel that your abdominals are creating a controlled arc of the spine so that the front of your body can roll without any jerkiness.

Reach the toes to the ceiling

Keep holding around the front of the feet

Arms stay straight

Arch the back with control

Thighs stay lifted off the mat

Chest stays lifted

Take care...

Make sure the arms pull evenly. You need to have even pressure on each foot to keep the rocking centered.

Do not compress the lower back. The spine should have an even curve, with the upper back opening as much as the lower back. Move the spine and limbs as one flowing unit. Set the movement going, and it should feel as if the movement could continue effortlessly, like a swinging pendulum.

What not to do

Don't pull your feet unevenly

Body is unbalanced

15-Minute Sequence

1 **The Hundred**
pp.144–145

2 **Roll Over**
pp.146–147

5 **Seal**
pp.158–159

6 **Saw**
pp.162–163

9 **Teaser 1**
pp.170–171

10 **Rocking**
pp.176–177

3 Double Straight Leg Stretch
pp.152–153

4 Criss-cross
p.154

7 Swan
pp.164–165

8 Double Leg Kick
pp.166–167

30-Minute Sequence

1 **The Hundred**
pp.144–145

2 **Roll Over**
pp.146–147

3 **Climb a Tree**
pp.148–149

7 **Open Leg Rocker**
pp.156–157

8 **Corkscrew**
pp.160–161

9 **Seal**
pp.158–159

13 **Teaser 1**
pp.170–171

14 **Teaser 2**
pp.172–173

15 **Rocking**
pp.176–177

4 Double Straight Leg Stretch
pp.152–153

5 Criss-cross
p.154

6 Spine Stretch Forward 3
p.155

10 Saw
pp.162–163

11 Swan
pp.164–165

12 Double Leg Kick
pp.166–167

16 Footwork 1
p.150

45-Minute Sequence

1 The Hundred
pp.144–145

2 Roll Over
pp.146–147

3 Climb a Tree
pp.148–149

7 Spine Stretch
Forward 3
p.155

8 Open Leg Rocker
pp.156–157

9 Corkscrew
pp.160–161

13 Double Leg Kick
pp.166–167

14 Scissors
pp.168–169

15 Teaser 1
pp.170–171

19
Footwork 2
p.151

4 Single Leg Stretch 2
p.100

5 Double Straight
Leg Stretch
pp.152–153

6 Criss-cross
p.154

10 Seal
pp.158–159

11 Saw
pp.162–163

12 Swan
pp.164–165

16 Teaser 2
pp.172–173

17 Teaser 3
pp.174–175

18 Rocking
pp.176–177

Assess your progress

How did you progress over the last six weeks? Go back and check your baselines (see pp.142–143). How do you feel compared to the first time that you performed the exercises? Did you notice an improvement? If so, well done! Keep at it!

Common problems

Did you make less progress than you'd hoped? Don't be disheartened. The challenges in this final section represent some of the most difficult and intense mat exercises in the Pilates repertoire. It can take people years to master them. They constantly offer more challenges, even if you have practiced for decades. This is the beauty of Pilates—there are always aspects to improve. If you truly take Pilates into your life, you will feel inspired and awed by the continuing challenge. Remember to review principles and key techniques as you exercise. If you are having difficulty, study the method and it will benefit your practice. Here are some common problems that you might face at this stage.

"I'm not enjoying this level; I feel 'stuck' and it's too difficult."

Pilates is tough! Try not to lose focus. If you're finding it hard to link many challenging exercises, mix and match the levels. Replace the exercises you're particularly struggling with in your workout by taking a few similar exercises from the Start Simple (see pp.26–87) and Build On It (see pp.88–139) chapters. That way, you will continue to build strength while working within your comfort zone. Aim to extend beyond your comfort zone ultimately, but take it slowly, introducing one or two extra exercises at a time. It will be easier to sustain your exercise program in the long-term if you link exercises from each level of the book in a balanced program that you feel suitably challenges your body.

"I'm disappointed because I don't have the body I wanted by this stage."

Perhaps your expectations were unrealistic. Pilates is wonderful for body conditioning, making you feel energized, toned, and inspired. However, if losing weight was your main aim, think about also modifying your diet and incorporating more cardiovascular exercise into your Pilates workout schedule. Monitor yourself to see how your body is changing to give yourself some encouragement. Measure the waist, upper arms, and upper thighs. After six weeks, measure them again. You might not have lost weight, but you should certainly have lost some inches and your appearance should be dramatically enhanced by a greater muscle tone and definition.

"I find The Hundred impossible and not at all fun!"

You're not the only one! Often there are groans when I teach this in class. It's a shame, since it can be a beautifully light and controlled exercise and is very effective at warming up the body and combining all Pilates principles (see pp.8–11). If your focus is not right, it can be labored, strained, and heavy. When attempting The Hundred, or any exercise that you find difficult, change your mindset. Instead of dreading it, be excited about the challenge. Think about bringing lightness and ease to the exercise. Imagine the head being gently lifted and the legs suspended lightly, rather than hanging from your pelvis. Your breathing is strong and even; the arms beat swiftly and fluidly, without rocking the spine and causing tension. Change your mental approach and you'll soon begin to love The Hundred!

Assess your achievement

Didn't achieve your goals? Don't lose your inspiration. Celebrate every achievement as you practice, for example being able to lift up smoothly into a Teaser 2 (see pp.172–173) or to roll your spine with more control in Roll Over (see pp.146–147). Small achievements accumulate—soon you'll be continually setting yourself new goals for the future.

Challenging exercises

Here is a plan to help you during your workouts over the next six weeks. At the end of the six weeks, look back over these goals and assess how you have progressed.

Goal: Control
Corkscrew (see pp.160–161)

Work on flowing the circular movement precisely and smoothly, without tension

Goal: Centering
Scissors (see pp.168–169)

Work on lengthening the legs from a strong core; keep the spine strong and supported

Goal: Flexibility
Open Leg Rocker (see pp.156–157)

Work on straightening the legs directly to the ceiling; keep the spine lengthened and rolling evenly on the mat

Goal: Strength
Teaser 1, Teaser 2, Teaser 3 (see pp.170–175)

Work on staying strong through the sequence, flowing each exercise to the next without a break

Goal: Flowing Movement
Rocking (see pp.176–177)

Work on rocking smoothly and evenly, without stopping and starting

The Future

I hope you've enjoyed this program and feel inspired to continue with Pilates. From now on, think about your goals and what areas you want to focus on as you exercise. Mix exercises from each level to keep up your interest and challenge your muscles afresh. Good luck!

Index

About the Author

Anya Hayes is a Pilates instructor based in London, and has been practicing Pilates for over 10 years. Anya trained with the world-renowned Body Control Pilates in London, and is passionate about restoring her clients' natural fluid movement and bringing them greater well-being. In her teaching Anya always hopes to inspire her clients with the amazing benefits that Pilates presents for body and mind, for all ages and fitness levels. Anya is a member of the Body Control Pilates Association (BCPA) and The Register of Exercise Professionals (REPS). She is the author of *My Pilates Guru*, and lives in London with her husband and baby son Maurice. Find her blog at http://memoandjoepilates.wordpress.com.

Acknowledgments

Photographic Credits

Dorling Kindersley would like to thank **Peter Anderson** and **Dave King** for new photography. All images © Dorling Kindersley. For further information see www.dkimages.com

Author's Acknowledgments

There are many people who deserve thanks for ensuring that this book came into existence. Firstly, to the wonderful teaching team at Body Control Pilates in London, where I trained, who are a continual source of inspiration for the never-ending learning on my own Pilates journey. To my fantastic teachers over the years, in particular Victoria Hodgson at Body Control and Deborah Henley at The Pilates Room, for encouraging me to push my own body and understanding to its limits and beyond in order to strengthen and progress. Thanks also to my lovely husband, and to my family for looking after the baby so I could write this book! Thanks to the DK editorial and design team for their patience and diligence in bringing the book to its completion.

Publisher's Acknowledgments

Many people helped in the making of this book. Dorling Kindersley would like to thank:

In the UK

Design assistance Vicky Read
Editorial assistance Annelise Evans, Kathryn Meeker
DK Images Claire Bowers, Freddie Marriage, Emma Shepherd, Romaine Werblow
Indexer Chris Bernstein

In India

Assistant Art Editor Tanya Mehrotra
Senior Art Editor Ranjita Bhattacharji
Design assistance Karan Chaudhary, Devan Das, Simran Kaur, Anchal Kaushal, Prashant Kumar, Ankita Mukherjee, Anamica Roy, Mahipal Singh, Vandna Sonkariya
Editors Vibha Malhotra, Kokila Manchanda
DTP Designers Rajesh Singh Adhikari, Sourabh Chhallaria, Arjinder Singh
CTS/DTP Manager Sunil Sharma